ENDOCRINE & METABOLIC
EMERGENCIES

Endocrine & Metabolic Emergencies

STEPHEN HAMBURGER, M.D.
Edward Hashinger Professor of Medicine
Chairman, Department of Internal Medicine
University of Missouri—Kansas City
Kansas City, Missouri

DAVID R. RUSH, B.S., PHARM. D.
Associate Professor of Medicine
  and Clinical Pharmacy
University of Missouri—Kansas City
Schools of Medicine and Pharmacy
Kansas City, Missouri

GIDEON BOSKER, M.D.
Member, Columbia Emergency Medicine Associates (CEMA)
Department of Emergency Medicine
Good Samaritan Hospital & Medical Center
Portland, Oregon

Robert J. Brady Co., Bowie, Maryland, 20715
A Prentice-Hall Publishing and Communications Company

Editor-in-Chief: David Culverwell
Acquisitions Editor: Richard A. Weimer
Production Editor: Janis K. Oppelt
Art Director: Don Sellers, AMI
Assistant Art Director: Bernard Vervin
Text Designer: Michael Rogers

Cover Art: Lynda J. Barry, Seattle, Washington
Indexer: Lea Kramer
Typesetter: Automated Graphic Systems, White Plains, Maryland
Printed By: R. R. Donnelley & Sons Co., Harrisonburg, Virginia

Endocrine & Metabolic Emergencies

Library of Congress Cataloging in Publication Data

Hamburger, Stephen , 1946–
    Endocrine & metabolic emergenices.

    Includes bibliographies and index.
    1. Endocrine glands—Diseases—Treatment.   2. Metabolism
—Disorders—Treatment.   3. Medical emergencies. I. Rush,
David R., 1946–   II. Bosker, Gideon,   III. Title.
IV. Title: Endocrine and metabolic emergencies.
[DNLM: 1. Emergencies.   2. Endocrine diseases.
3. Metabolic diseases. WK 100 H1995e]
RC649.H295   1984   616.4'025   83-22334
ISBN 0-89303-436-3

Prentice-Hall International, Inc., London
Prentice-Hall Canada, Inc., Scarborough, Ontario
Prentice-Hall of Australia, Pty., Ltd., Sydney
Prentice-Hall of India Private Limited, New Delhi
Prentice-Hall of Japan, Inc., Tokyo
Prentice-Hall of Southeast Asia Pte. Ltd., Singapore
Whitehall Books, Limited, Petone, New Zealand
Editora Prentice-Hall Do Brasil LTDA., Rio de Janeiro

Printed in the United States of America

84 85 86 87 88 89 90 91 92 93 94   10 9 8 7 6 5 4 3 2 1

CONTENTS

PREFACE

Emergency medicine, as a specialty, has grown significantly in the past few decades. By definition, the clinical practice of this field interfaces with other disciplines, particularly internal medicine. Within internal medicine, endocrine and metabolic emergencies are relatively infrequent but, in most instances, highly treatable with a good prognosis. It is our intention that *Endocrine & Metabolic Emergencies* will bring to the reader diagnostic strategies and treatment plans for this interesting and challenging subspecialty which bridges the fields of internal and emergency medicine.

ACKNOWLEDGMENTS

Just as "no man is an island unto himself," no book is just the editor/authors to themselves. We would like to take this opportunity to express our sincere thanks and appreciation to Sue Blake, Stephanie Etheridge, Pat Zetocka and Gayle Kelley for their expertise in secretarial assistance, and to Jean Sarkis for her time and energy in aiding the authors in their library searches. We gratefully acknowledge the contributions of Alexis Thomas, M.D. and Jean Otrakji, M.D. for their chapters on sodium and potassium disorders, respectively.

DEDICATION

To LIH, JVH, and MSH with love and admiration

To Raymond and Helen Rush with love

You are the bows from which your children as living arrows are set forth

Kahil Gibran (1883–1931)
The Prophet, "On Children"

1

DIABETIC KETOACIDOSIS (DKA)

INTRODUCTION

Diabetes mellitus is a common illness in the United States. Although the significant morbidity and mortality associated with diabetes mellitus are secondary to the vascular long-term complications, at least one acute manifestation of the illness, namely diabetic ketoacidosis (DKA), is deemed a classic, life-threatening, medical emergency. Its formerly high mortality rate has been drastically reduced by recent developments in diagnosis and management. Although considerable knowledge has accumulated in the various aspects of its therapy, there is still an approximately 5 to 10 percent mortality rate in most medical centers. In select subgroups such as the elderly patient, the mortality rate may be significantly higher.

General Considerations

Diabetic ketoacidosis may be defined as a state of relative or absolute insulin deficiency which results in an excessive ketone concentration (beta-hydroxybutyrate [BHB], acetoacetate [AcAc], and acetone), a low bicarbonate concentration, and a low arterial pH. Hyperglycemia is usually present.

DKA is one of the most common acute medical disorders encountered by the emergency physician. It requires immediate diagnostic and therapeutic intervention, along with precise laboratory and clinical monitoring. Fortunately, with the availability of insulin, a former metabolic catastrophe resulting in a high mortality rate has become an emergency that can be resolved if detected early and treated appropriately with fluids, electrolytes, and insulin. Most deaths are due to concomitant coronary artery disease with or without myocardial infarction, infection, renal failure, cerebrovascular disease, or other causes. A diligent search to detect precipitating factors is imperative in DKA, but usually this evaluation cannot be accomplished within the province of the emergency department.

Etiology

Diabetic ketoacidosis may be either the mode of initial presentation of the diabetic patient or an incident in the course of the disease. Precipitating factors in its acute development include the stress of general anesthesia and surgery, dehydration from fluid restriction or gastrointestinal disease, intercurrent infections, pharmacological doses of corticosteroids, and the accidental or deliberate omission of insulin.

DIAGNOSIS

Presentation

Clinically, hyperglycemia manifests as polyuria, polydipsia, malaise, and visual difficulties with resultant intravascular volume depletion. An osmotic diuresis leads to loss of sodium, potassium, magnesium, chloride, and phosphorus. The acidemic environment can precipitate many adverse neurologic, metabolic, respiratory, and cardiovascular effects. Abdominal pain, nausea, and vomiting frequently complicate the early course of DKA and can potentiate the volume depletion induced by the hyperglycemic diuresis. Aci-

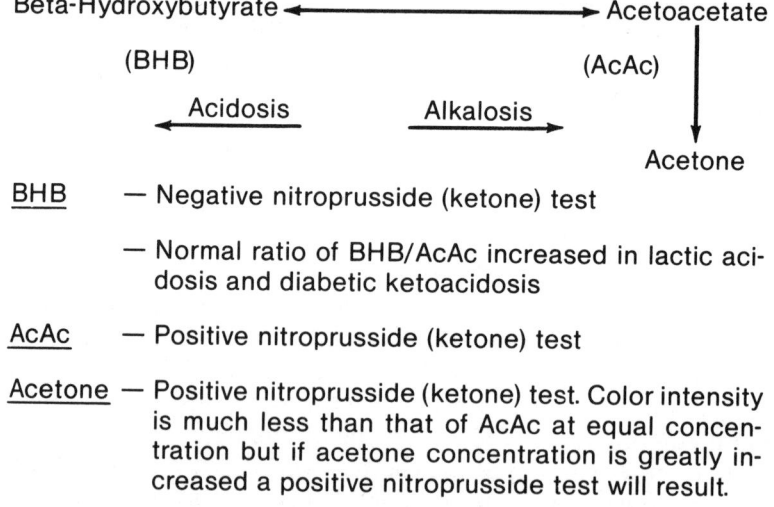

Beta-Hydroxybutyrate ⟷ Acetoacetate

(BHB)   (AcAc)

← Acidosis   Alkalosis →

Acetone

BHB — Negative nitroprusside (ketone) test

— Normal ratio of BHB/AcAc increased in lactic acidosis and diabetic ketoacidosis

AcAc — Positive nitroprusside (ketone) test

Acetone — Positive nitroprusside (ketone) test. Color intensity is much less than that of AcAc at equal concentration but if acetone concentration is greatly increased a positive nitroprusside test will result.

Figure 1–1. Nitroprusside Reaction.

TABLE 1–1.   COMMON PRECIPITATING FACTORS OF DKA

Failure of Endogenous Insulin	Previously undiagnosed diabetic Viral infections of pancreas Pancreatitis Idiopathic/autoimmune
Hormonal Antagonism of Insulin	Cushing's syndrome Thyrotoxicosis Pheochromocytoma Acromegaly
Failure of Exogenous Insulin	Change in diet or exercise Patient noncompliance • Inadequate patient education • Poor vision • Wrong insulin concentration • Calibration/injection error • Mental deficiency Inadequate dose or type prescribed Insulin antibodies
Stress	Infection (e.g., pneumonia, abscess, UTI, gangrene) Pregnancy Myocardial infarction Surgery Trauma Acute psychiatric illness
Drug Therapy	Thiazide diuretics Glucocorticoid steroids Dilantin

dosis is also responsible for one of the classic signs of DKA, rapid deep Kussmaul breathing. Tachypnea usually precedes Kussmaul breathing, which is an attempt to compensate for the metabolic acidosis of DKA by lowering arterial pCO_2. Usually this type of respiration is noted when the serum bicarbonate falls to near 10 mEq/liter; however, as the arterial pH falls below 7.1, the patient may lose his respiratory drive and thus lose this compensating mechanism.

An odor of decaying apples or "Juicy Fruit®" gum on the patient's breath is another classic sign of DKA; acetone is responsible for this odor. The odor may not be prominent in the DKA patient whose ketone production is markedly shifted toward HBHB. One practical point to remember: there is an excellent correlation between concentrations of breath acetone and plasma acetone.

The mental status of the DKA patient can vary from full alertness to drowsiness or deep coma. None of the standard measures of metabolic derangement in current use are predictive of the expected level of consciousness. The majority of patients will be conscious at time of presentation.

The severity of illness may vary widely. The patient is invariably hyperglycemic, usually hyperosmolar, and a positive nitroprusside reaction (e.g., Acetest®) is usually obtained. However, none of these reactions are prerequisites of DKA. The patient who has had severe vomiting with loss of hydrogen, potassium, and chloride ions or who has taken alkali may present with diabetic "ketoalkalosis" rather than classic DKA.

Many—but by no means all—patients presenting with clinical DKA have already been diagnosed as diabetics. The presenting symptoms of DKA can be quite variable. However, most of the symptoms can be explained by the defect in intermediary metabolism and the intravascular volume deficiency with poor tissue perfusion.

Patients presenting with DKA usually have a several-day history of the following symptoms:

- Increased urination and thirst secondary to the osmotic diuresis
- Increasing weakness and weight loss secondary to the catabolism of body fat and protein stores and anorexia, nausea, vomiting
- Variable mental symptomatology arising from the ketotic state and intravascular volume depletion.

In a known diabetic, these symptoms, when they occur in increasing severity, are highly suspect of DKA; otherwise a suspicion of DKA is one of clinical judgment. In fact, DKA should be uncommon in the known, compliant diabetic because the symptoms of DKA are usually present for several days prior to severe clinical and metabolic decompensation and should be recognized by the patient. Moreover, if the patient tests his urine for glucose and ketones properly, these tests will reflect a poor degree of control and alert him to the potential for DKA long before it actually develops.

Initial examination of the DKA patient must include a meticulous search to determine what events precipitated the metabolic decompensation. The most frequent causes are patient noncompliance and infection. In elderly patients especially, painless myocardial infarction may be present and a baseline EKG should be obtained in the emergency department to facilitate this diagnosis.

The adequacy of intravascular volume should be evaluated by measuring the blood pressure and pulse with the patient in the supine and erect positions if at all possible. Skin turgor, tissue perfusion, CNS symptoms, urinary output, and skin temperature should also be assessed.

The DKA patient with abdominal pain presents a special problem. Diabetic patients are not immune from surgical problems involving the gastrointestinal tract, but many will have the "pseudoappendicitis" of DKA. Although hyperamylasemia (and an elevated amylase/creatinine clearance ratio) is seen in a significant percentage of diabetic patients with DKA, most do not have acute pancreatitis. However, almost all patients with DKA have a leucocytosis (usually $15-20 \times 10^3/mm^3$) with a left shift. The leukemoid reaction in severe acidosis should be kept in mind when ruling out infectious causes of DKA.

Since abdominal signs and symptoms subside with treatment of the ketotic state, it is essential to correct the DKA as rapidly as possible to avoid unnecessary surgery. If, despite adequate treatment of DKA, abdominal signs and symptoms persist, a surgical condition should be considered. Recent studies suggest that any patient over age 40 with DKA and abdominal pain is likely to have an underlying problem causing the pain. Also, patients with abdominal pain who have a serum bicarbonate level greater than 10 mEq/liter are likely to have an underlying condition producing their abdominal pain. However, it must be stressed that underlying conditions producing abdominal pain are frequently of medical (i.e., gastroenteritis, etc.) rather than of surgical origin.

Laboratory

Initial Diagnostic Strategy

When DKA is suspected, laboratory tests that should be carried out immediately include:

- Clinistix® or Diastix® test for urinary glucose
- Acetest with undiluted serum for ketones
- A complete arterial blood gas analysis.

Any patient with strongly positive ketones, 4+ glycosuria, a low arterial pH resulting from a primary metabolic acidosis, and correlating clinical findings is in DKA and should be treated accordingly.

Laboratory Evaluation

While the patient's history and physical data are being gathered, additional laboratory evaluation should be initiated. Appropriate work-up of the patient with DKA includes serum glucose, electrolytes, BUN/creatinine, osmolality, ketone bodies, CBC, phosphate, magnesium, and other tests as indicated. Since quantitative plasma ketone measurements are not routinely available or their results are delayed, you should rely on the qualitative nitroprusside reaction. The nitroprusside in Acetest does not react with BHB and reflects only the concentration of AcAc (and, to a lesser extent, acetone). If, as is often the case in DKA, there is an increased degree of tissue hypoxia with an ensuing increase in lactic acid, the BHB/AcAc ratio is shifted further to favor BHB. This is secondary to the increased level of NADH that results from tissue hypoxia. Thus, it is important not to miss or underestimate the severity of ketoacidosis if there is a negative, trace, or weakly positive nitroprusside reaction.

Finally, appropriate gram strains and cultures should be done to rule out infection.

Special Diagnostic Considerations

Electrolytes and BUN

Interpretation of the serum sodium must take into account the "pseudohyponatremia" induced by hyperglycemia. For every 100 mg% elevation of glucose above 100, the serum sodium is reduced by 1.6 mEq/ml. Knowledge of this relationship is important in determining the water deficit in such a patient. Hyperlipidemia or hyperproteinemia can also cause an artificial hyponatremia, since the large lipid or protein molecules present occupy a significant portion of the total serum volume that is analyzed for sodium concentration.

Tests of kidney function may be misleading because the BUN, which is almost always high, may have a significant pre-renal component in its increase, and the creatinine may be spuriously elevated by the AcAc if the colorimetric method of determination is used. Arterial blood gases reflect a pure metabolic acidosis with a respiratory compensation in uncomplicated DKA. You should suspect superimposed lactic acidosis if the nitroprusside test is weakly positive in the presence of a significant acidemic state and an elevated anion gap.

$$\text{Anion Gap} = (Na^+) - (Cl^- + HCO_3^-) = 12 \pm 2 \text{ mEq/L}$$

Nitroprusside Reaction

As mentioned, the nitroprusside reaction measures AcAc and, to a much lesser extent, acetone; it does not measure BHB, even in large concentrations. In a normal person, the BHB/AcAc ratio is approximately 2/1. Acidemia will shift this equilibrium to BHB, while alkalemia does the reverse. In DKA, the BHB/AcAc ratio is increased to approximately 3/1, though cases in which the ratio is as high as 30/1 have been documented.

The nitroprusside reagent is only 1/20 as sensitive to acetone as it is to AcAc; thus, the nitroprusside reaction is only a qualitative estimation of the total ketone concentration.

Drawbacks to unquestioning reliance on the nitroprusside reaction are seen in a subset of patients with DKA, i.e., those who are susceptible to the simultaneous development of lactic acidosis secondary to their severe hypovolemic state or underlying cardiovascular disease. It has been estimated that these two disorders occur concomitantly in up to 30 percent of patients. Lactic acidosis shifts the BHB/AcAc ratio to BHB, which makes the nitroprusside reaction negative or less reactive. The simultaneous occurrence of lactic acidosis can produce an underestimation of the severity of the ketoacidosis by the nitroprusside reaction.

With adequate volume expansion and insulin therapy, the ketoacidosis and lactic acidosis will resolve rapidly. In most cases of uncomplicated DKA, the acidotic state will correct within 12–24 hours. With correction of the abnormal acid-base balance, the BHB/AcAc ratio shifts to AcAc. In a small series of patients it has been shown that the AcAc concentration remains unchanged or may increase during early treatment. Because of its slow excretion and metabolization, the acetone concentration may remain elevated for as long as 42 hours after treatment is begun. In addition, an acetone concentration of greater than 5 mM, present in many patients with DKA, may produce a positive nitroprusside reaction. For these reasons, it is possible either to have a prolonged positive nitroprusside reaction or to see a reaction become strongly positive during successful treatment of DKA. However, careful clinical and laboratory monitoring will put the nitroprusside reaction into proper perspective.

MANAGEMENT

General Considerations

The therapy of diabetic ketoacidosis must be individualized and emphasizes the following:

1. Vigorous replacement of fluid and electrolyte deficits
2. Normalization of intermediary metabolism with insulin
3. Diagnosis and treatment of any precipitating event(s)
4. Avoidance of complications
5. Education of the patient so that recurrences will be minimized.

In regard to correction of the intermediary metabolism, there is no clear evidence that any route of low-dose insulin therapy is clearly superior, and, therefore, the clinician should be comfortable with both the intramuscular and intravenous routes.

Therapeutic Measures

Volume replacement

Emergency treatment begins with prompt intravenous administration of saline solution, even before the results of initial biochemical determinations (plasma levels of glucose and electrolytes, and blood ph) are available. Restoration of the extracellular fluid volume is the mainstay of emergency management for patients with DKA and is the single most important ingredient in the success of any insulin regimen.

The average patient will require about 6–8 liters of normal and/or half normal saline during the first 24 hours of treatment of severe DKA. Whether normal or half normal saline is used depends on the status of the intravascular volume and serum osmolality. The intravascular volume, which is most easily corrected by normal saline, is measured by following criteria of volume repletion such as blood pressure, pulse, neck vein distention, mentation, skin temperature and urine output. Use of a central venous pressure (CVP) line is discouraged unless clearly indicated. If indicated, Swan-Ganz monitoring may be more appropriate. During intravascular volume repletion, the patient must be constantly monitored not only for adequacy of volume replacement but also for symptoms and signs of sodium overload such as hypertension or congestive heart failure.

Serum glucose may fall significantly with volume expansion alone, sometimes by as much as 20 percent. Thus, the early fall in plasma glucose levels must be cautiously interpreted in the face of simultaneous volume repletion and insulin administration. Continuous monitoring of plasma glucose levels will identify a sustained drop. Initial values should include measurement of the plasma osmolality as this number will help guide water replacement. Plasma osmolality may be estimated by the formula below:

$$2(Na+) + glucose/18 + BUN/2.8$$

Most patients with DKA will have some degree of increased plasma osmolality due to hypotonic urinary loss. With repletion of the intravascular volume by saline solutions and lowering of the plasma sugar by insulin, much of the hyperosmolality will be corrected. If the plasma osmolality is still elevated, the use of hypotonic fluids such as half normal saline or free water by mouth will lower the osmolality. Rapid correction of the free water deficit is undesirable as it has not been shown to be clinically beneficial and might be potentially harmful in regard to producing cerebral edema.

In all cases of well established DKA, there exists a significant total body depletion of sodium and water. Estimated sodium loss is approximately 8–10 mEq/kg and water 75–100 ml/kg of body weight. Losses occur principally from the osmotic diuresis, as well as vomiting and diarrhea.

In addition, insulin directly stimulates renal tubular reabsorption of sodium. Thus, the deficiency of insulin in DKA may cause additional renal wasting of sodium. Studies have shown that the urinary output in DKA resembles half-normal saline with 35–63 mEq/liter of potassium. Regardless of this hypotonic urinary loss, serum sodium levels in untreated DKA are mostly low or normal. This may occur secondary to the "pseudohyponatremia" induced by hyperglycemia. For every 100 mg percent elevation of glucose above 100 mg%, the serum sodium is reduced by 1.6 mEq/ml. In calculating the water deficit in a patient with DKA, this relationship must be known. An elevation in serum triglycerides may result in factitious hyponatremia. A normal or increased serum osmolality coupled with a low serum sodium suggests this possibility. An elevated uric acid level may occur secondary to decreased renal perfusion and competitive inhibition of uric acid secretion in the distal renal tubule by the ketone bodies or by lactic acid.

Insulin Therapy

Diabetic ketoacidosis is caused by a relative or absolute deficiency of insulin, resulting in a profound defect in intermediary metabolism. This deficiency produces two major metabolic abnormalities: hyperglycemia and hyperketonemia. The former is secondary to overproduction of glucose from glycogenolysis and gluconeogenesis and underutilization of glucose. The latter has two major components: overproduction and underutilization of ketoacids. Optimal insulin therapy in diabetic ketoacidosis is achieved when sufficient levels are delivered to peripheral target tissues (liver, adipose tissue and muscle) in order to reverse these metabolic deficiencies and simultaneously minimize the risk of adverse insulin-induced effects such hypoglycemia, hypokalemia, hypophosphatemia, and cerebral edema. The maximum effect of insulin in diabetic ketoacidosis is achieved with circulating concentrations of approximately 20 to 200 uU/ml. Complete hepatic inhibition of glucose production usually occurs with insulin concentrations between 100–200 uU/ml. Maximum peripheral glucose uptake requires an insulin concentration of approximately 200 uU/ml although concentrations below this level will produce a significant glucose pickup. Insulin inhibition of lipolysis requires a considerably lower concentration, approximately 30 to 50 uU/ml, while the metabolism of ketoacids is achieved with an insulin concentration of between 50–100 uU/ml. Successful therapy of diabetic ketoacidosis with circulating insulin levels of approximately 100 uU/ml suggest that high physiologic rather than pharmacologic concentrations are important. Adequate concentrations of insulin have been readily achieved by intramuscular, intravenous, and subcutaneous routes of administration.

By various routes and protocols, low-dose insulin therapy has been employed with great effectiveness in the emergency treatment of diabetic ketoacidosis. Once the diagnosis of DKA is confirmed, insulin therapy should be initiated immediately. The following routes of administration are recommended—intramuscular and low-dose intravenous.

Intramuscular.   Convenient to administer and rapidly acting, low-dose intramuscular insulin has been used with great effectiveness in the treatment of diabetic ketoacidosis. Intramuscular insulin has a half life of about two hours. An initial injection of 20 units of regular insulin followed by 10 units per hour intramuscularly will result in an insulin concentration of approximately 100 uU/ml in less than 3 hours. In the adequately volume-repleted patient, the plasma glucose will fall by about 100 mg/dl per hour; there will be a commensurate fall in the level of blood ketones. Using an initial intramuscular dose of 0.1 uU/lb body weight and 5–10 units of regular insulin IM per hour thereafter, the plasma glucose will usually correct to 250 mg/dl in approximately 6–8 hours. Correction of the arterial pH ($[HCO_3] \geq 20$ mmol/L) usually occurs several hours after the response of the plasma glucose. Patients who fail to demonstrate at least a 10 percent fall in plasma glucose by the end of the first hour should receive a repeat loading dose every hour until a 10 percent decline in plasma glucose has been achieved. A minority of patients in which the intramuscular route is employed will require a repeat priming dose.

Although the intramuscular route predictably lowers plasma glucose by 70–100 mg/dl per hour and restores plasma pH, aggressive volume repletion (see page 7) is a prerequisite for achieving these therapeutic endpoints in patients with diabetic ketoacidosis.

Correction of the ketoacidosis takes a few hours longer than restoration of the plasma glucose; the slower correction of the acidosis is acceptable, since a precipitous elevation of arterial pH may result in profound hypokalemia, hypophosphatemia, shifts in the oxyhemoglobin dissocation curve, and neurologic abnormalities. Generally, hypoglycemia and hypokalemia are less frequent with low-dose intramuscular regimens than with high-dose insulin therapy. As with other low-dose insulin regimes, patients with underlying infection will have a slower decline in their plasma glucose. The recommended site of injection is the deltoid muscle. If low dose intramuscular insulin is chosen, the following regimen is recommended:

In the adequately volume-repleted patient:

1. Use the deltoid muscle.
2. Administer 0.1 unit/lb of body weight of regular insulin as an initial dose. Use no less than 10 units of regular insulin.

3. If the plasma glucose fails to decrease by 10 percent in the first hour, repeat priming dose; repeat priming dose each hour thereafter until a 10 percent decrease in plasma glucose is obtained.
4. If an adequate plasma glucose response is obtained with the initial dose, begin 0.05 units/lb body weight of regular insulin (no less than 5 units) each hour until plasma glucose is approximately 250 mg/dl.
5. If there is no response in the plasma glucose after 3 doses, switch to intravenous continuous insulin and search vigorously for an infection.
6. An intravenous loading dose (with step 2) of 0.05 units/lb of body weight of regular insulin is optional. (Use between 4 and 8 units.) If there is any doubt concerning the practicality of using a continuous insulin infusion, the intramuscular route of insulin administration is the treatment of choice.

Low-Dose Intravenous.   The success of continual low-dose insulin therapy in the treatment of diabetic ketoacidosis has been well established. Low-dose intravenous infusion of insulin readily achieves a circulating concentration (i.e., 100 uU/ml) adequate for reversal of metabolic defects. A priming (i.e., loading) dose of 2 to 12 units of regular insulin intravenously followed by 5 to 10 units/hour constant infusion is sufficient to reduce plasma glucose by 75 to 100 mg/dl per hour. Using this method, hyperglycemia and ketoacidosis can usually be corrected within 10 hours.

As with low-dose intramuscular insulin, intravenous therapy is generally associated with less hypoglycemia and hypokalemia than non-continuous high dose therapy. Because insulin binds with glass and plastic, many centers recommend the use of human albumin, a gelatin solution, or addition of the patient's own blood to the insulin solution to prevent adsorption. Although of theoretical importance, the clinical significance of the adsorption is doubtful; several studies have shown excellent results with low-dose intravenous insulin therapy in the absence of any binding inhibitor. Nevertheless, if an inhibitor is not added, the "washout" technique should be employed. By running 100 ml of a solution containing 5.0 U/dl or greater of regular insulin through the tubing before connecting to the patient, potential insulin binding sites will be occupied, allowing maximum insulin delivery. Bolus intravenous therapy is discouraged as insulin levels will fluctuate from early pharmacological levels to suboptimal concentrations before the next dose is given. As with intramuscular insulin therapy, infected patients seem to respond slower. If constant intravenous insulin infusion is chosen for treatment of diabetic ketoacidosis, the following is recommended:

In the adequately volume-repleted patient:

1. Use the "washout" technique prior to connecting the insulin infusion to patient.
2. Begin continuous regular insulin infusion of 7 units per hour until plasma glucose is 250 mg/dl.
3. If no response is achieved with step 2:
   a. Double insulin infusion rate
   b. Search diligently for an infection
   c. Add binding inhibitor.
4. An intravenous loading dose of regular insulin (3 to 5 units) is optional.

It should be stressed that the goal of insulin therapy in diabetic ketoacidosis is correction of the ketotic state. Thus, the aim of any route of insulin therapy is not to see how low a dose may be administered but to achieve an adequate concentration of insulin to reverse the metabolic abnormalities. If intravenous therapy is chosen, optimal results are observed with an infusion rate of 4–10 units of regular insulin per hour.

Subcutaneous route.   Although low dose subcutaneous insulin has been used successfully in diabetic ketoacidosis, other routes of insulin therapy have been more fully scrutinized and are probably preferable to subcutaneous administration.

Complications of Insulin Therapy

Hypoglycemia

By any method of administration, insulin may induce hypoglycemia. With low-dose insulin therapy, the drop in blood glucose is predictable, and with frequent monitoring of the blood sugar, this complication should be infrequent. As the blood sugar approaches 250 mg percent, exogenous glucose should be added either by vein or orally. It is important to realize that as the exogenous sugar is added, insulin will still need to be given but the dosage and route of administration may have to be adjusted. The correction of the acidosis tends to lag behind the normalization of the blood sugar but as long as improvement in the pH is shown, this delay should be of little concern.

Cerebral Edema

Fortunately cerebral edema is very uncommon, but a frequent fatal complication of DKA. Suspicion of this complication should occur in any patient in whom clinical and biochemical improvement is followed by deterioration in cerebral function. Elevation of the intraocular or CSF pressures (with or without papilledema) in such a patient strongly suggests this complication. Although no treatment is of proven benefit, free water administration should be stopped and hypertonic saline or mannitol begun in hope of reversing the process.

Clinically, most cases of cerebral edema occur in patients whose blood sugars are reduced rapidly to normal. Cerebral edema is uncommon when the blood sugar is not lowered rapidly to below 250 mg percent. Thus, in the management of DKA, the early supplementation of exogenous sugar (at approximately 250 mg percent) and less reliance on markedly hypotonic solutions to correct the increased serum osmolality should reduce the frequency of this complication.

Alkali Therapy

Alkali therapy in DKA remains controversial. Weighing the benefits and risks, it is clear that alkali should be used in very few cases of DKA. Although indications for alkali infusion are not firmly established, sodium bicarbonate (44 to 88 mEq, 1 to 2 ampules) IV should be administered to patients with DKA who have:

1. An arterial pH of 7.10 or less
2. Significant cardiac arrhythmias associated with a low arterial pH
3. Hypoventilation secondary to severe acidosis.

The latter may be suggested by an abnormal elevation of the pCO_2, according to Winter's formula in a primary compensated metabolic acidosis.

$$\text{Expected } pCO_2 = 1.54 \, (HCO_3-) + 8.34 \pm 1.1$$

If the pCO_2 is higher than expected, a mixed acid-base disturbance (metabolic and respiratory acidosis) is occurring. Very infrequently (usually at a pH of about 6.8) the hypoventilation may be secondary to acidemic depression of the breathing center. In any case, the alkali of choice is bicarbonate. Therapy should be given to correct the pH to no higher than 7.20 and a bicarbonate level of about 10 mEq/liter. The latter assures some margin of safety if the process worsens. If used, bicarbonate therapy should be slowly infused and its effect on arterial pH frequently monitored. Caution should be used in the use of alkali therapy as no study has shown a clear benefit of its use and several groups have reported no difference or a possible negative effect when alkali is included in the treatment.

Complications.   Alkali therapy is not without risk. In untreated ketoacidosis, the oxyhemoglobin dissociation curve approximates a normal p_{50} (arterial oxygen-tension at which 50 percent of hemoglobin is oxygenated).

This near normal p_{50} is due to the counterbalancing effect of acidosis and the low 2,3-diphosphoglyceric acid (2,3-DPG). A too rapid or overcorrection of the acidemic state may shift the oxyhemoglobin dissocation curve to the left producing tissue hypoxemia secondary to the increased binding of oxygen by hemoglobin. In addition, alkali therapy has been shown to accentuate the intracellular shift of potassium and phosphate.

To maintain normal concentration of potassium and phosphate, exogenous administrations of these substances may need to be increased. Hypophosphatemia has been shown to have several deleterious effects including myocardial depression, white blood cell abnormalities, central nervous system dysfunction, and insulin resistance. Also, injudicious use of alkali in DKA is associated with "paradoxical" cerebrospinal fluid acidosis. Because of the different permeability of the blood brain barrier to CO_2 and HCO_3, rapid correction of the acidosis with alkali therapy will cause an accentuated drop in cerebrospinal fluid pH which normally occurs during therapy. In addition, this "paradoxical" intracellular acidosis may occur in other organ systems. The clinical consequences of this "paradoxical" acidosis is largely unknown, but one study suggests a detrimental effect on neurological function. Lastly, alkali therapy has been frequently associated with tetany secondary to the shift of calcium or magnesium or both to the albumin-bound form.

Potassium Therapy

In the absence of known hyperkalemia or ECG changes of hyperkalemia, appropriate potassium administration, in the form of potassium chloride or possibly potassium phosphate, is indicated along with volume replacement and insulin therapy. If the potassium level is elevated, potassium should be withheld until the plasma concentration is in the high normal range. Oliguria and renal failure are relative contraindications to potassium administration.

With the initiation of therapy, for DKA, plasma potassium falls rapidly, usually to its lowest level within four hours. The decline in the potassium level is secondary to numerous factors including rehydration, insulin-induced uptake of potassium by cells, and the shift of potassium within cells as the acidosis is corrected. In addition, up to 50 percent of the exogenous potassium administered may be lost in the urine.

To maintain a normal potassium concentration, approximately 100 to 150 mEq of potassium may have to be given in the first few hours. Potassium therapy in all patients must be closely monitored by frequent blood samples. The use of ECG for sequential monitoring of prevailing plasma potassium levels is discouraged.

Magnesium Therapy

DKA is associated with a significant urinary loss of magnesium. As with potassium, the initial magnesium level might be normal or high but tends to drop with initiation of insulin and fluid therapy. Clinical symptomatology of hypomagnesemia is similar to hypocalcemia and includes tetany, seizures, cardiac arrhythmias, and central nervous system depression. A serum magnesium level should be drawn upon presentation and, if low, magnesium should be administered preferably by vein. This is particularly true in the early therapy of DKA as the intramuscular pickup might be less than optimal until adequate intravascular volume has been achieved. In the presence of seizures or arrhythmias of uncertain etiology, magnesium therapy should be considered even if the magnesium level is normal. Magnesium should be administered very cautiously, if at all, in renal insufficiency. Frequent blood levels should be checked as should the deep tendon reflexes of the patient. As magnesium levels rise to toxic concentrations, deep tendon reflexes diminish. Magnesium replacement should be accomplished by the IV or IM route; the IV route should be reserved for patients requiring immediate control of seizures or tetanic contractions. When this method is employed, 1–2 grams of magnesium sulfate as a 10 percent solution should be given over 15–30 minutes.

Special Therapeutic Considerations

Hypophosphatemia

Etiology.   Phosphate depletion in diabetic ketoacidosis arises from many sources. Most patients have anorexia and a good percentage will have vomiting or diarrhea or both. Thus, there will be decreased phosphorous intake and increased intestinal loss of phosphorous. Glycosuria, ketonuria, and polyuria are associated with excessive renal loss of phosphorous, while hypomagnesemia, another common abnormality in diabetic ketoacidosis, may also produce excessive renal phosphate wasting. Although all of these mechanisms are not operative simultaneously, there is a significant loss of total body phosphorous with estimates ranging from 1mM per kg of body weight to 400 mM.

Clinical derangements in pronounced phosphorus depletion may involve:

1. Tissue oxygenation
2. Neutrophil function
3. Central nervous system function
4. Glucose utilization.

Phosphorus therapy.   Although nearly all patients have a total body depletion of phosphorous, only a small proportion of patients

TABLE 1–2.   MECHANISMS OF PHOSPHOROUS LOSS IN DIABETIC KETOACIDOSIS

Increased Intestinal Loss	Vomiting
	Diarrhea
Increased Renal Loss	Acidosis
	Glycosuria
	Renal tubular defects
	Hypomagnesemia
	Hypokalemia
	Metabolic alkalosis
Intracellular Shift	Treated diabetic ketoacidosis
	Respiratory alkalosis

will have hypophosphatemia at the time of diagnosis. However, serum phosphate levels and urinary excretion of phosphorous and serum phosphate levels will decrease dramatically in the first few hours of insulin therapy. A plasma phosphate concentration below 1.0 mg/dl, which may occur commonly in diabetic ketoacidosis, has potentially serious consequences on body metabolism and organ function and is an indication for immediate phosphorus therapy.

Therapeutic guidelines for phosphorous administration in the treatment of severe hypophosphatemia are few and mainly empiric. Although oral phosphate preparations are available, parenteral administration is recommended for the pronounced phosphate depletion state. An initial dose of 0.08 mmol/kg body weight (2.5 mg/kg body weight) is recommended if hypophosphatemia is recent and uncomplicated; 0.16 mmol/kg body weight (5 mg/kg body weight) if it is prolonged and has multiple causes. Initial doses should be 25 to 50 percent higher if the patient is symptomatic or if serum phosphate level is less than 0.8 mg/dl. Each dose should be given intravenously over a period of six hours. Because these guidelines are empiric, the effect of therapy must be closely monitored.

Complications.   Phosphorous administration is not without hazard. Depending on which phosphate sale is given, hypernatremia and its attendant complications or hyperkalemia may occur. Both symptomatic hypocalcemia and hypomagnesemia have been well documented during phosphate therapy; thus, clinical symptoms and biochemical values for these electrolytes should be closely watched. Metastatic calcification may occur and deterioration of renal function is relatively common. In addition, rapid administration of phosphorous may cause severe hypotension. Contraindications to phosphorous administration include hyperphosphatemia, hypomagnesemia, hypocalcemia, and renal insufficiency. Oral phosphorous solutions may produce diarrhea.

REFERENCES

Cryer PE, Daughaday WH: Diabetic ketosis elevated serum glutamic-oxal-oacetic transaminase (SGOT) and other findings determined by multi-channel chemical analysis. Diabetes, Vol 18, No 781, 1969

Fisher JN, Shahshahnani MN, Kitabchi AE: Diabetic ketoacidosis: Low-dose insulin therapy by various routes. N Engl J Med, Vol 297, No 238, 1977

Kitabchi AE, Ayyagari, V, Guerra SMD: The efficacy of low-dose versus conventional therapy of insulin for treatment of diabetic ketoacidosis. Ann Intern Med, Vol 84, No 633, 1976

Knight AH, Williams DN, Ellis G, et al: Significance of hyperamylasaemia and abdominal pain in diabetic ketoacidosis. Br Med J, Vol 3, No 128, 1973

Knight AH, Williams DN, Spooner RJ, et al: Serum enzyme changes in diabetic ketoacidosis. Diabetes, Vol 23, No 126, 1974

Kreisberg RA: Diabetic ketoacidosis: New concepts and trends in patho-genesis and treatment. Ann Intern Med, Vol 88, No 681, 1978

Levine RL, Glauser FL, Berk JD: Enhancement of the amylase-creatinine clearance ratio in disorders other than acute pancreatitis. N Engl J Med, Vol 292, No 329, 1975

Sherwin R, Felig P: Pathophysiology of diabetes mellitus. Med Clin North Am, Vol 62, No 695, 1978

Sulway MJ, Malins JM: Acetone in diabetic ketoacidosis. Lancet, Vol 2, No 736, 1970

Warshaw AL, Feller ER, Lee KH: On the cause of raised serum amylase in diabetic ketoacidosis. Lancet, Vol 1, No 929, 1977

2

HYPOGLYCEMIA

INTRODUCTION

General Considerations

Extreme downward deflections in plasma (or blood) glucose concentrations frequently present as a medical emergency. The diagnosis of hypoglycemia in acute situations is easily made when the blood glucose level is low. In non-acute cases, however, hypoglycemia can be difficult to diagnose because it is not a disease, but an indication of derangement in glucose homeostasis. Hypoglycemia may present with a wide spectrum of signs and symptoms—both emergent and non-emergent. The establishment of the diagnosis is made by documentation of a low blood glucose level associated with symptoms relieved by glucose administration.

A major area of dispute in hypoglycemia has been to define the lower limits of a "normal" blood glucose. Hypoglycemia in adults has been rather arbitrarily defined as occurring when the plasma glucose falls below 50 mg/dl (true whole blood glucose below 40 mg/dl). When such a reduction is accompanied by symptoms and signs of adrenergic hyperactivity or nervous system depression, or a combination of both, clinical as well as chemical hypoglycemia is manifest.

Much of the earlier literature attempting to define hypoglycemia at a specific circulating glucose level is confusing since often there was no differentiation between blood glucose and serum glucose. Blood glucose levels are generally 7 to 9 mg/dl lower than serum levels because of the volume dilution effect of red blood cells. The defining of an arbitrary cutoff blood glucose level to represent hypoglycemia has been complicated both by the inexact defining of measurements by investigators and the finding that blood glucose levels below 50 mg/dl are not always accompanied by clinical symptoms. Recent data has also shown that normal females in a 72-hour fasting state may have plasma glucose levels 10 mg/dl lower than their male counterparts.

Certainly, these figures are confusing in defining the allowable lower limits of blood glucose. The conditions preceding these tests certainly can affect the conclusions. In these and other studies, conditions preceding the tests vary from an overnight fast or prolonged fast to simply looking at the reactive glucose nadir.

Despite all these inconsistencies of findings and definitions some practical operative guidelines are necessary. Five general guidelines are offered for the diagnosis of hypoglycemia:

1. In adult males and females a random blood sample drawn in association with hypoglycemic signs and symptoms, a plasma glucose below 50 mg/dl (blood glucose less than 40)
2. In adult males and females after an overnight fast, a plasma glucose below 60 mg/dl (blood glucose less than 52)
3. In adult males fasted for 72 hours, a plasma glucose below 55 mg/dl (blood glucose less than 47)
4. In adult females fasted for 72 hours, a plasma glucose less than 45 mg/dl (blood glucose less than 40)
5. In adult males and females given a 100-Gm oral glucose load, lowest plasma glucose less than 55 mg/dl (blood glucose less than 47).

Pathophysiology

It is important to understand the basic physiologic considerations that make hypoglycemia so important to recognize, classify, and treat. The brain is uniquely vulnerable to acute depletion of circulating glucose. Failure to recognize the clinical condition may result in irreversible damage to neural cells, which may lead to permanent impairment of mental function, personality, and motor and sensory nerve functions.

The brain's most important substrate for energy metabolism is glucose. Under normal conditions, 90 percent of the oxidative metabolism is sustained by combustion of glucose. The brain is dependent on a constant supply of glucose from the blood circulation since the brain's carbohydrate deposits can compensate for only a few minutes of utilization. The transportation of glucose from the blood to the nerve and glial cell metabolic apparatus of the brain involves a number of steps. These include:

- Transport through the blood-brain barrier
- Diffusion through the extra-cellular space of the brain
- Transport through nerve and glial cell membranes
- To a lesser degree, transport over the choroid plexus.

Whether the action of insulin on brain glucose metabolism plays any role under physiological conditions is unclear at present. Despite the fact that insulin plays a major role in the regulation of glucose transport and metabolism in the human body, the hormone appears to have no direct effect on the transport mechanisms for glucose across the blood-brain barrier. While our present knowledge indicates insulin has no direct action on glucose transport from blood to brain, by means of its influence on glucose metabolism, the net transport of glucose from blood to the brain is certainly augmented by insulin.

There are three major pathways through which the brain obtains glucose:

1. Glucose homeostasis in the fed state is due primarily to glucose absorbed from the intestinal tract. The complex carbohydrates which generally comprise 50 percent of the typical Western world diet are hydrolyzed to simple monosaccharides within the lumen of the gut and the intestinal brush border. Glucose (80 percent) is the major component of this breakdown along with fructose (15 percent) and galactose (5 percent). The glucose and galactose are actively transported to blood via a carrier-mediated system of the intestinal cells and provide the most direct potential substrate for the brain.

2. The utilization of hepatic (and to a much lesser degree, renal) glycogen

3. The catabolization of proteins and amino acids to glucose.

The last two pathways are utilized to maintain glucose homeostasis primarily in the postabsorptive phase of a meal (4 to 6 hours after eating) or during more prolonged fasting.

The liver, which is freely permeable to glucose and does not require insulin for glucose transport, takes up approximately 50 percent of the splanchnic glucose transport. This is then phosphorylated via glucokinase under insulin control. Most of the assimilated carbohydrate is converted to glycogen. Its storage in the liver makes this organ an important depot for glucose. During fasting between meals, or under stress situations, hepatic glycogen is the primary substrate for maintaining circulating glucose concentrations. Prolonged fasting depletes hepatic glycogen stores and the normal 25 percent contribution of gluconeogenesis to keeping glucose levels normal may, of necessity, approach 100 percent.

Hepatic glycogen content is normally 80 to 100 grams. While an additional 400 grams of glycogen is stored in the muscle, only the liver portion can be rapidly converted to glucose. Hepatic glycogen reserves can be diminished within 24 to 48 hours during fasting to only a 10 gram reserve for acute stresses.

The nervous system, mainly the brain, requires about 100 mg of glucose per minute to insure proper functioning. The 144 grams per day required for the brain alone exceeds the total glycogen stored in the liver at any one time. As outlined above, hepatic glycogen stores are maintained during fasting by gluconeogenesis as "new" glucose is made available by the conversion of amino acids from protein or from incompletely oxidized substrates such as lactic acid. Thus, to prevent the development of hypoglycemia, all three pathways for providing circulating glucose to the brain are very important.

DIAGNOSIS

In recent years, hypoglycemia has been popularized by the lay press as the basis for a diversity of human ailments. Hypoglycemia has been characterized as a nondisease of epidemic proportions. Because of the unwarranted proliferation of the hypoglycemia diagnosis, the American Diabetes Association, American Medical Association, and the Endocrine Society jointly published a "Statement on Hypoglycemia" that cautioned against attributing a number of unrelated diseases to hypoglycemia. Several studies have looked at the link between depression, anxiety, hypochondriacal and hysterical personality features, and the hypoglycemia diagnosis. It appears that many patients with symptoms of hypoglycemia also have emotional disturbances, however, there is no support for a cause-and-effect relation between the two conditions.

A number of classification systems have been proposed for hypoglycemia based on physiologic mechanisms, mode of clinical presentation, or the organic systems involved. The most common physiologic approach is to characterize the hypoglycemia as either fasting (spontaneous) hypoglycemia, postprandial (post absorptive reactive) hypoglycemia, or toxic hypoglycemia. The major advantage to this system is that it facilitates a more logical and practical approach to diagnosis and treatment. A general outline of this approach is presented in Table 2–1.

Clinical Presentation

Clinical manifestations of hypoglycemia are usually not manifest until the plasma glucose falls below 50 mg/dl. As has already been mentioned, there is a poor correlation between symptomatology and corresponding levels of circulating glucose. Some patients are entirely asymptomatic with plasma glucoses of less than 50 mg/dl. Additionally, it is often observed that neuroglucopenic symptoms of hypoglycemia may tend to persist for a time even after extracellular glucose levels have returned to normal.

TABLE 2-1. CLINICAL CLASSIFICATION OF HYPOGLYCEMIA

Fasting Hypoglycemia (Spontaneous)
Pancreatic Beta Cell Tumors (Insulinoma) or Hyperplasia
- Adenoma, single or multiple (90%)
- Carcinoma (10%)
- Nesidioblastosis (in infants and children)

Extra Pancreatic Tumors [Insulin Secreting and Nonsuppressible insulin-like activity (NSILA-s)]
- Mesenchymal (40–60%)
- Hepatoma (20–25%)
- Andrenocortical carcinoma (5–10%)
- Gastrointestinal (5–10%)

Endocrine Hypofunction (Counter-Insulin Glucoregulatory Hormones)
- Anterior Pituitary Hypofunction
    Panhypopituitarism
    Growth Hormone Deficiency
    ACTH Deficiency
- Deficient Counter-Insulin Glucoregulatory Hormones
    Glucocorticoid Deficiency
    Thyroid Insufficiency
    Glucagon Insufficiency
    Catecholamine Deficiency
- Adrenocortical Hypofunction

Acquired Diffuse Hepatic Dysfunction
- Acute Hepatic Necrosis
    Viral
    Hepatotoxin
    Refractory Congestive Heart Failure (rare)

Congenital Hepatic Disorders (Gluconeogenesis Disorders)
- Glyconeogenic Enzyme Deficiences
- Glycogen Metabolism Disorders

Substrate Limitations
- Alanine Deficiency (Infant Ketotic Hypoglycemia)
- Defective Substrate Conversion
- Pregnancy
- Severe Deficiency of Nutrient Intake (Inanition)
- Renal Failure

Insulin Autoimmune Hypoglycemia

Postprandial Hypoglycemia (Postabsorptive Reactive)
Alimentary
- Partial or Total Gastrectomy
- Gastrojejunostomy
- Vagotomy and Pyloroplasty
- No Gastrointestinal Surgery
    Increased Gastric Emptying
    Abnormal Intestinal Glucose Absorption

TABLE 2–1.   CLINICAL CLASSIFICATION OF HYPOGLYCEMIA (continued)

Idiopathic Hypoglycemia
Developing Diabetes Mellitus
Glactose—Induced
Fructose—Induced
Leucine—Induced

Pharmacologic and Toxic-Induced Hypoglycemia
Insulin
Sulfonylureas   Iatrogenic or Factitious
Ethanol
Propranolol, Salicylates, and other miscellaneous drugs
Ingestion of ackee fruit (hypoglycin)

Signs and Symptoms

The clinical picture of hypoglycemia is protean. However, the symptoms and signs of hypoglycemia in the adult can be divided into those due to adrenergic nervous system activation and those due to altered cortical and subcortical function. They are outlined in Table 2–2.

The activation of the sympathetic nervous system is more likely to occur with the rapid decline in extracellular glucose. However, it appears that not only the rate of decline but also the breakthrough of a low glucose threshold may trigger the sympathetic discharge. This threshold is probably repetitive in the same patient along with the sequencing of manifestations and patterns of recurrence, but the threshold appears to clinically vary from subject to subject.

The first factor to recognize about hypoglycemia is that it is episodic in nature. While the symptoms may recur repeatedly, ongoing symptoms of chronic fatique or personality aberrations that last for days or weeks should not be attributed to hypoglycemia. With true hypoglycemia one of three outcomes usually results within minutes to hours:

1. Normal counter-regulatory mechanisms are activated and the blood glucose level reverts to normal
2. Intake of dietary glucose sources results in normal blood glucose levels
3. Or, if neither of the above occur, the blood glucose level continues to fall resulting in progression of signs and symptoms of neuroglucopenia.

Insulin-Induced Hypoglycemia

The most common cause of hypoglycemia encountered in practice is the self-administration of exogenous insulin. Most of these patients are diabetics and the recognition that hypoglycemia epi-

TABLE 2–2.   SIGNS AND SYMPTOMS OF HYPOGLYCEMIA

Adrenergic Activation	*Disturbed Cortical Function*
Beta Stimulation	Weakness
• Tremulousness	Headache
• Tachycardia	Blurred or Double Vision
• Palpitations	Disturbed Intellectual Function
• Diaphoresis	Amnesia
• Faintness	Incoordination or Paralysis
Anxiety	Seizures
Hunger	Coma
Gastric Hypermotility	Brain Stem Dysfunction
Nausea	

sodes are very common among insulin-dependent patients is necessary to prevent hypoglycemic sequelae. If the physician is unsure as to whether neuro-psychiatric signs, including coma in the diabetic patient, are resulting from relative insulin excess or hyperglycemia due to diabetic ketoacidosis or hyperosmolor nonketotic coma, parenteral glucose should be given immediately after obtaining blood for glucose analysis. Less cerebral damage is likely to occur from the administration of glucose erroneously to a hyperglycemic patient than would occur if glucose was withheld from a hypoglycemic patient. An error of commission is much preferable to one of omission in this situation.

"Factitious" Hypoglycemia

Occasionally, particularly among health care workers, clandestine use of insulin may result in "factitious" hypoglycemia. These patients can be best identified by the finding of insulin and syringes on their person or by additional laboratory work-up. The key finding is an absent or low plasma C-peptide in the face of a low glucose and high insulin levels. This virtually excludes the presence of endogenous hyperinsulinism. The C-peptide is a portion of the proinsulin molecule that is split off when insulin is secreted and can be detected by radioimmunoassay. Exogenously administered insulin does not result in high C-peptide levels along with high insulin levels thus C-peptide can serve as a marker for endogenous insulin. In the chronic abuser of insulin, the detection of the presence of circulating insulin antibodies would also support the diagnosis.

Somogyi Effect

Another consideration in insulin-induced hypoglycemia is the change, over time, from a typical hypoglycemic response associated with a warning phase predominated by autonomic discharge to an atypical insulin reaction devoid of autonomic nervous system signs or the appearance of these only at greatly elevated glucose levels. Additionally, the occurrence of occult nocturnal hypoglycemia followed by early morning glucose level elevations in the insulin-treated diabetic is of practical concern. This Somogyi effect may be suspected if there is a history of nightmares, night sweats, nocturnal diaphoresis, sleep disturbances, or early morning headaches with a "hungover" feeling. Several objective tests can help establish this entity. Certainly a nighttime glucose (i.e., 1–3 A.M.) showing hypoglycemia would be helpful. A quantitative urine glucose determination for the 12 midnight to 6 A.M. interval would generally be the lowest in comparison to the other six-hour samples collected during the day. The use of urinary free cortisol determination performed on the morning urine sample can also be helpful if it is excessively elevated.

Correction of this problem may be achieved by decreasing the morning intermediate or long-acting insulin and replacing a portion of it with regular insulin. If an evening dose is being given, it should be reduced or eliminated. A regular bedtime snack consisting of both carbohydrate and protein should be prescribed for all patients on intermediate or long-acting insulin.

Hypoglycemia Secondary to Oral Hypoglycemic Agents

Hypoglycemia can also arise in the patient on oral sulfonylurea compounds or those taking them surreptitiously. Glucopenic reactions to the oral hypoglycemics may be much more profound and hazardous than those to insulin because of the long duration of their presence and physiologic effect. Chlorpropamide appears to have the highest incidence of hypoglycemic reactions. The factitious use of these agents complicates ruling out the laboratory diagnosis of insulinoma. It is often necessary to screen blood and urine for the presence of these compounds if they are suspicioned. In addition, with the occurrence of hypoglycemia in a patient on oral hypoglycemic agents a concerted effort should be made to rule out drug-drug interactions that may have yielded a potentiation of the hypoglycemic effect. Among the many agents that have been reported to cause this effect, ethanol, salicylates, oral anticoagulants, and phenylbutazone are probably the most significant. These same interacting drugs along with other compounds such as beta adrenergic blockers, sulfonamides, chloramphenicol, chlorpromazine, and monoamine oxidase inhibitors have been cited as causes of glucopenia.

Ethanol-Induced Hypoglycemia

A final common etiologic agent in the production of pharmacologic hypoglycemia is ethanol consumption. Ethanol itself is not a primary hypoglycemic agent. However, in the setting of glycogen stores depletion due to prolonged poor intake of carbohydrate and excessive alcohol intake, hypoglycemia can occur. Ethanol-induced changes in glucose metabolism have been identified that lead to inadequate gluconeogenesis and glucose release. This entity presents primarily in alcoholics who have been drinking for several days at a time.

Additionally, alcohol can enhance insulin release after glucose ingestion and has been reported to contribute to postprandial hypoglycemia. It has also been postulated that alcoholic drinks with glucose-containing mixers are more apt to produce this type of hypoglycemia than are straight alcohol drinks. Any patients prone to hypoglycemia or receiving any form of hypoglycemic treatment should be warned of the inherent dangers of alcohol overindulgence.

Fasting Hypoglycemia

Physiologically, fasting hypoglycemia occurs as a result of decreased gluconeogenesis, impaired glycogenolysis from the liver, or a combination of both. An organic etiology is usually demonstrated with the major causes of fasting hypoglycemia being:

1. Excessive circulating insulin or insulin-like substances due to insulinomas, pancreatic hyperplasia, or extra pancreatic tumors secreting insulin or non suppressible insulin-like compounds
2. Counter-insulin glucoregulatory hormone deficiencies and endocrine hypofunction
3. Congenital or acquired hepatic dysfunction
4. Substrate limitations.

Simply stated, hypoglycemia occurring spontaneously in the fasting state can be due to either an underproduction of glucose or an overutilization of glucose.

Deficient glucose production can be due to disorders of glycogen metabolism or storage, or impairment of gluconeogenesis due to substrate defects of limitations. As these forms of glucopenia occur primarily in infants or children and are relatively rare in occurrence, they will not be discussed.

Deficiencies of counterinsulin glucoregulatory hormones can lead to fasting hypoglycemia. The specific hormones of primary interest in this neuroendocrine control system are catecholamines, glucagon, glucocorticoids, growth hormone and thyroid hormones. In part, they oppose the anabolic actions of insulin. Also these hormones counter the action of insulin during the transition from the fed to the fasting state and meet energy demands by combinations of the following:

1. Direct stimulation of the pathways of glycogenolysis and gluconeogenesis to augment hepatic glucose output

2. Inhibition of glucose uptake and assimilation of insulin-sensitive tissues
3. Inhibiting insulin release
4. Providing glucogenic substrate
5. Mobilizing alternative energy sources.

Table 2–3 outlines the physiologic actions of counterinsulin hormones and the relative roles each plays in the control system. Deficiencies in secretion of glucagon, epinephrine and norepinephrine, cortisol and thyroid hormones although all working by several mechanisms result primarily in decreasing hepatic gluconeogenesis. Growth hormones' major action appears to be in decreasing insulin activity in the peripheral tissues.

Insulinoma

Excessive secretion of insulin by B-cell tumors of the pancreas may cause hypoglycemia by overutilization of glucose. Ninety percent of these tumors are benign adenomas; 10 percent are malignant carcinomas which most often metastasize to the liver and regional lymph nodes. The nonspecific triad (symptomatic, fasting hypoglycemia reversed by glucose) is generally the first suspicion of hyperinsulinism. The diagnosis is frequently unsuspected for years since the symptoms are often intermittent, nonspecific, and insidious in onset and progression. Eventually, the actions of insulin counterregulatory hormones and the adaptation of insulin receptors to high levels of circulating insulin are overcome and this partial protection to the effects of an insulinoma is lost. There is rarely, however, a dramatic isolated episode of hypoglycemia just a slow progression of the disorder.

The oral glucose tolerance test shows an erratic response in such patients. Protraction of this test to 6–12 hours may dramatically demonstrate hypoglycemia as protracted fasting can exacerbate the disorder. Vigorous physical exercise can also make the symptomatology more evident. Confirmation of the suspected diagnosis necessitates the confirmation of insulin levels that are inappropriately elevated for a low plasma glucose.

The ratio of plasma insulin to glucose (microunits per ml/mg per 100 ml) has been used to quantitate the insulin and glucose relationship. The normal patient has a ratio below 0.25 while the insulinoma patient ratio is generally above 0.40. An index has also been proposed to substantiate the same thing. It is determined by:

$$\frac{\text{Plasma insulin } (\mu\text{U/ml}) \times 100}{\text{Plasma glucose } (\text{mg}/100 \text{ ml}) - 30}$$

Levels greater than 50 are indicative of insulinoma. C-peptide levels are also inappropriately elevated in patients with insulinomas. A test on these levels in insulin-treated diabetics with circulating

TABLE 2–3. PHYSIOLOGIC ACTIONS OF COUNTERINSULIN HORMONES*

	Insulin Release	Muscle Glucose Uptake	Hepatic Gluconeogenesis	Proteolysis	Lipolysis	Ketogenesis
Epinephrine and Norepinephrine	↓	↓	↑	↑	↑	↑
Glucagon	—	—	↑	—	—	↑
Cortisol	—	—	↑	↑	↑	↑
Growth Hormone	—	↓	—	↓	↑	↑
Thyroid Hormones	—	—	↑	↑	↑	↑

* ↑ = increase
↓ = decrease
— = no major effect

insulin antibodies suspected of having an insulinoma is very helpful.

Pharmacologic provocative tests to evoke excessive release of insulin have been well described. Tolbutamide, glucagon, and leucine have all been used but are not usually necessary. These tests all have a certain degree of risk and an attendant number of false-positive and false-negative results.

Nonsuppressible insulin-like activity substances (NSILA-s) and extra-pancreatic tumors have also been identified as etiologic agents in hypoglycemia. While increased glucose assimilation by the tumor might theoretically occur, it appears that the tumors may induce hypoglycemia by producing a factor that influences glucose homeostasis. One such factor is NSILA-s. These substances have been isolated in the presence of low circulating insulin levels and may themselves be the hypoglycemic factor rather than insulin. Additional work may clarify the role of these substances and their relationship with hypoglycemia.

An autoimmune origin for hypoglycemia has been described where there are high serum insulin levels and antibodies to insulin. However, the binding of antibody to hormone may be altered such that free insulin is released unexpectedly at inappropriate times leading to hypoglycemia.

Other Causes

Hypopituitarism and hypoadrenocorticism can lead to decreased gluconeogenesis and fasting hypoglycemia. Hypoglycemia during exercise may be a common presentation in childhood hypopituitarism. Often this entity presents as a seizure with associated low blood glucose and low plasma insulin levels. Growth hormone or glucocorticoids are usually successful in these disorders.

TREATMENT

Acute Hypoglycemia

The approaches to treatment of hypoglycemia are simple. Administration of glucose is the main thrust of treatment. Serious fasting or insulin-induced hypoglycemia producing confusion, neuro-psychiatric impairment, or coma is best treated by the intravenous administration of a bolus of 25 to 50 grams of glucose as a 50 percent solution followed by a continuous infusion of 5–10 percent (or greater) glucose until the patient is able to eat. It is important to remember that hepatic glycogen repletion is not accomplished by the initial glucose administration. Meal intake is a therapeutic endpoint whereupon intravenous glucose administration may be discontinued. Spontaneous hypoglycemia due to endocrine hypofunction may additionally require hormone replacement. In chronic alcoholics and other individuals susceptible to thiamine deficiency, 100 mg of thiamine should be administered intramuscularly to prevent acute Wernicke's encephalopathy.

If the patient's swallowing mechanisms are intact and the hypoglycemia is manifest primarily by an adrenergic reaction without neuroglucopenic signs, simple oral carbohydrates (i.e., glucose-containing liquids) can be given. Parenteral therapy would be preferred, however, if there is any predisposition to possible aspiration. Therapy of recurrent hypoglycemia is dietary. Often, simple avoidance of fasting is all that is required.

The use of intramuscular injections of 1 mg of glucagon usually is not necessary in the hospital setting where intravenous glucose administration is so easily accomplished. However, this form of treatment at home by nonmedical personnel is still warranted, particularly in the patient at risk of insulin-induced toxic hypoglycemia.

Toxic hypoglycemia due to sulfonylureas may persist for days. This is particularly true with chlorpropamide and its active hepatic metabolites and prolonged elimination in renal disease. These patients often require extended periods (days) of glucose infusion as they can lapse back into coma if the glucose is stopped prematurely. Indeed, such a patient with prolonged overutilization of glucose may best have their glucose administration titered to achieve a mild degree of glycosuria. The persistence of the oral hypoglycemic activity may be due to its inherent long serum half-life and variable metabolism and elimination in patients with hepatic or renal compromise.

Chronic Hypoglycemia

In the patient with true insulinoma, surgery is the treatment of choice. Celiac or superior mesenteric arteriography is usually done to try to localize the lesion. If the tumor is not palpated in the pancreas, a stepwise tail to head pancreatectomy is carried out with intraoperative analysis of sequential frozen sections. Analysis of pancreatic vein insulin concentrations and frequent plasma glucose measurements can be helpful. An abrupt increase in plasma glucose during surgery may indicate excision of the tumor. Surgery is usually stopped when 85 percent of the pancreas has been removed to avoid postoperative malabsorption complications. The use of streptozotocin, mithramycin, and adriamycin in the treatment of unresectable or metastatic insulin-producing carcinomas has had limited success. Streptozotocin has provided the best palliative results via systemic or celiac artery injection. Diazoxide has been used intravenously or orally in 0.3–1.2 gm per day doses prior to surgery and in post-operative care where the tumor was not isolated. This drug reduces the release of insulin and may be helpful but usually requires the concomitant use of a diuretic to combat its salt-retaining properties.

Postprandial Hypoglycemia

There are many situations in which the hypoglycemia occurs only in response to some stimulus. The most common stimuli is food intake. The terms functional, reactive, or postprandial hypoglycemia have been used to identify this group of disorders and to contrast them with hypoglycemias occurring in the fasted state. Patients with such "functional" hypoglycemia have normal fasting blood glucose concentrations but become hypoglycemic 30 minutes to four hours after a carbohydrate-containing meal. In this situation the blood glucose concentration may fall below 50 mg per 100 ml but does not progress to coma or brain stem dysfunction. Complaints are predominately those of adrenergic activations.

These symptoms are generally not caused by fasting or exercise but can be precipitated by an oral five-hour glucose tolerance test. While this is the most widely used test for establishing the diagnosis, the levels of plasma glucose considered to be abnormal during the second to fifth hours of the test are quite controversial. Even though levels of 50 mg per 100 ml or below have been suggested as being abnormal, this level is debated since normal subjects often reach even lower levels without concomitant symptoms. Those with early glucose nadirs on the oral glucose tolerance test are classified as alimentary in origin while those with late nadirs are often reflective of early diabetes.

While the hypersecretion of insulin has been demonstrated in some individuals after a high carbohydrate-containing meal, this is a very variable response. The pre-diabetics often secrete insulin more slowly than normal but for a more extended duration resulting in hypoglycemic levels hours after the glucose load is given.

Initial treatment is aimed at minimizing the stimulus for insulin secretion. Patients with postprandial hypoglycemia often receive relief of their symptoms by avoiding refined carbohydrate loads and by changing to a high protein, low-carbohydrate diet. Cholinergic blocking agents have also been used with some success.

Alimentary hypoglycemia is a postprandial phenomenon (90 to 180 minutes after meals) that commonly occurs as an accepted complication after various gastrointestinal surgeries including partial or total gastrectomy, gastrojejunostomy, or pyloroplasty. While some investigators include alimentary hypoglycemia as one of the common complications of the "dumping syndrome," itself postgastrointestinal surgery, others define it as an associated but separate complication of gastric surgery.

The patient with true alimentary hypoglycemia may respond to multiple small meals. Diets high in complex carbohydrate and fiber and low in simple sugars have generally replaced low-carbohydrate diets. Propranolol, although still investigational for this use, may be an effective adjunct to dietary therapy. The mechanism for this effect of propranolol is not yet clear.

Failure to maintain the plasma glucose concentration within its relatively narrow limits can lead to a critical situation. In the short run hypoglycemia represents a greater risk as a metabolic abnormality than does hyperglycemia. Glucose is the primary energy substrate of the brain and must be maintained at a normal constant level to avoid the cellular complications of hypoglycemia and brain cell death itself.

Apart from insulin reactions in diabetics, hypoglycemia has not been a common problem in the practice of medicine. The diagnosis or "label" of postprandial hypoglycemia has been made with great unrestricted frequency in recent years. Definitions of these disorders and methods of appropriate diagnosis and treatment are imperative for the practicing physician.

REFERENCES

Cahill GF, Soeldner JS: A non-editorial on non hypoglycemia. New England Journal of Medicine, Vol 291, pp 905–906, 1974

Cole RA, Benedict GW, Margolis S, Kowarski A: Blood glucose monitoring in symptomatic hypoglycemia. Diabetes, Vol 25, pp 984–988, 1976

Ensinck JW, Williams RH: Disorders causing hypoglycemia. In Williams RH (ed): Textbook of Endocrinology, 6th ed. W. B. Saunders Co., Philadelphia, Pennsylvania, pp 844–875, 1981

Fajans SS, Floyd JC: Diagnosis and medical management of insulinomas. Annual Review of Medicine, Vol 30, p 313 1979

Fajans SS, Floyd JC: Fasting hypoglycemia in adults. N Engl J Med, Vol 294, 766–772, 1976

Felig P: Disorders of Carbohydrate Metabolism, In Bondy PK, Rosenberg LE (eds): Metabolic Control and Disease, 8th ed., W.B. Saunders Co., Philadelphia, Pennsylvania, 1980

Ford CV, Bray GA, Swerdloff RS: A psychiatric study of patients referred with a diagnosis of hypoglycemia. Am J Psych, Vol 133, pp 200–294, 1976.

Gastineau CF: Is reactive hypoglycemia a clinical entity? Mayo Clinic Proceedings, Vol 58, No 8, pp 545–549, August 1983

Hofeldt FD: Reactive hypoglycemia. Metabolism, Vol 24, pp 1195–1208, 1975

Hogan MJ, Service FJ, Sharbrough FW, et al: Oral glucose tolerance test compared with a mixed meal in the diagnosis of reactive hypoglycemia: A caveat on stimulation. Mayo Clinic Proceedings, Vol 58, No 8, pp 491–496, August 1983

Johnson DD, Dorr KE, Swenson WM, Service J: Reactive hypoglycemia, JAMA, Vol 243, pp 1151–1155, 1980

Leichter SB: Alimentary hypoglycemia: A new appraisal. Am J Clin Nutr, Vol 32, pp 2104–2114, 1979

Merimee TJ, Tyson JE: Hypoglycemia in man, Diabetes, Vol 26, pp 161–165, 1977

Miller DR, Bolinger RE, Janigan D, et al: Hypoglycemia due to non-pancreatic mesodermal tumors. Annals of Surgery, Vol 150, pp 684–696, 1959

Seltzer HS: Drug-induced hypoglycemia. Diabetes, Vol 21, pp 955–960, 1972

Shen SW, Bressler R: Hypoglycemia. Rational Drug Therapy, Vol 11, pp 1–6, 1977

Somogyi M: Exacerbation of diabetes by excess insulin action. Diabetes, Vol 13, pp 600–605, 1964

Special Report from the American Diabetes Association. The Endocrine Society and the American Medical Association: Statement on Hypoglycemia Diabetes, Vol 22, No 137, 1973

Turner RC, Oakley NW, Nabarro JDN: Control of basal insulin secretion with special reference to the diagnosis of insulinomas. Brit Med J, Vol 2, pp 132–135, 1971

Yager J, Young RT: Non-hypoglycemia is an epidemic condition, N Engl J Med, Vol 291, pp 907–908, 1974

3

HYPEROSMOLAR HYPERGLYCEMIC NONKETOTIC COMA (HHNK)

INTRODUCTION

The clinical syndrome of diabetes mellitus encompasses several medical emergencies, the most prominent of which are diabetic ketoacidosis (DKA), and hyperosmolar hyperglycemic nonketotic coma (HHNK). HHNK has become a frequently recognized complication of diabetes mellitus. Although HHNK was initially described nearly a century ago, awareness of this syndrome has increased in recent years. Despite increased recognition of this syndrome, which is characterized by pronounced hyperglycemia, hyperosmolality and dehydration in the absence of ketoacidosis, the mortality rate remains significantly higher than that of DKA even in patients of comparable age. Many fatalities are attributable to a delay in diagnosis and initiation of appropriate therapy.

Pathogenesis

Although pathogenetic mechanisms in the syndrome of HHNK have not been completely elucidated, interest in its pathogenesis has focused on the lack of significant ketosis and depressed sensorium. Ketone bodies are normally produced by the liver in proportion to the circulating levels of free fatty acids (FFA) which act as substrate. Several reports have revealed that the FFA levels in HHNK are either normal or less than those found in DKA, implying a defect in lipolysis. Lipolysis depends on many variables including

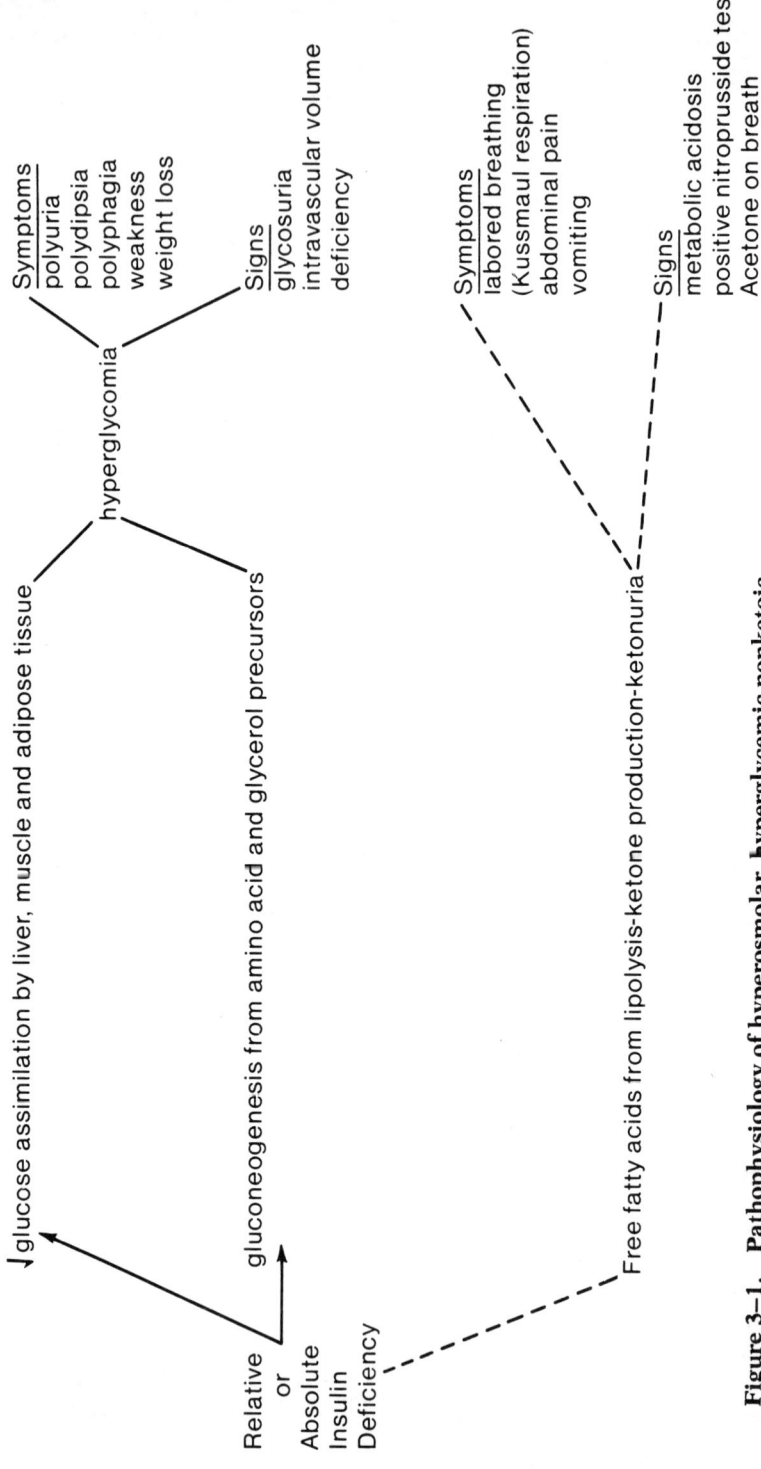

Figure 3–1. Pathophysiology of hyperosmolar, hyperglycemic nonketoic coma (HHNK). In HHNK the broken lines are suppressed.

the circulating levels of insulin, growth hormone, and cortisol, all
of which may modulate the release of FFA from adipose tissue.
Although the circulating levels of insulin have been found to be
similar in patients with HHNK and DKA, growth hormone and
cortisol, lipolytic hormones, have been found to be significantly
lower than in patients with DKA. These results suggest that in some
patients with HHNK the low levels of FFA and lack of ketosis might
reflect the lower activity of lipolytic hormones. Other mechanisms
for the lack of ketosis in this syndrome have been postulated. It has
been suggested that severe dehydration might be antiketogenic
resulting in low plasma FFA levels and ketone production, while in
vitro studies have revealed that hyperosmolality inhibits the release
of pancreatic insulin to glucose and FFA production from adipose
tissue. Depressed sensorium in HHNK is correlated with the plasma
osmolality. Nearly stuporous or obtunded patients have a plasma
osmolality of at least 350 mOsm/kg where patients with a plasma
osmolality of less than 350 mOsm/kg usually are more alert. Sensorium does not correlate with the glucose concentration or the pH
of either cerebrospinal fluid or plasma.

Pathophysiology

Metabolic abnormalities, including osmotic shifts and renal
response mechanisms, determine therapeutic strategies in patients
with HHNK. The fundamental derangements in HHNK include a
relative lack of insulin and a relative excess of anti-insulin hormones including growth hormone, cortisol and glucagon (see Table
3–1). The net result of the interaction of these hormones is excessive
production and underutilization of glucose which results in pronounced hyperglycemia. Total body water generally represents about
60 percent of body weight with two-thirds of water being intracellular and one-third being extracellular. As the plasma glucose ele-
vates, water moves from the intracellular fluid to the extracellular
space until osmotic equilibrium is achieved. Thus pronounced
hyperglycemia results in the loss of water from the intracellular
fluid which produces intracellular dehydration and concomitant
albeit transient expansion of the extracellular fluid. These fluid and
electrolyte shifts have diagnostic and therapeutic implications. As
the plasma glucose rises, the renal threshold for glucose reabsorption is surpassed resulting in glycosuria. Generally, the higher the
glucose, the greater the renal excretion of glucose. Glycosuria causes
an osmotic diuresis by inhibiting the reabsorption of water which
results in increased urine flow. With respect to loss of electrolytes,
the osmotic diuresis in patients with HHNK is approximately 50
mEq sodium/liter, while urinary potassium losses are about the
same. The osmotic diuresis produces a water loss that is in excess
of sodium losses resulting in a hyperosmolar state and an intracel-

TABLE 3–1.   METABOLIC EFFECTS OF THE ANTI-INSULIN HORMONES

	Insulin Release	*Muscle Glucose Uptake*	*Gluconecogenesis*	*Lipolysis*
Glucagon	↑	↓	↑	↑
Growth hormone	↑	↓		↑
Glucocorticoids	↑	↓	↑	↑

lular water depletion in most patients with HHNK. In addition, the loss of sodium leads to depletion of extracellular fluid volume. Much of the hyperglycemia in the patient with HHNK results in part from decreased renal excretion of glucose as well as decreased cellular uptake. As the extracellular fluid volume becomes depleted, the glomerular filtration rate decreases, thus dampening the normal renal escape mechanism for glucose. Thus a vicious cycle occurs:

1. The higher the plasma glucose the more pronounced the depletion of extracellular volume
2. The glomerular filtration decreases
3. Less glucose is excreted in the urine
4. The plasma glucose becomes more elevated.

A similar circumstance has been shown to occur in patients with DKA where much of the hyperglycemia is secondary to impaired excretion of renal glucose. In addition to the urinary loss of sodium, potassium, and water, other electrolytes including magnesium and phosphate have also been found to be depleted in patients with HHNK. In most instances, patients with HHNK have more pronounced volume depletion and higher plasma glucose levels than patients with DKA because of longer duration of symptoms before therapy is initiated.

DIAGNOSIS

Clinical

HHNK occurs mainly in the elderly patient with an average age of 60 years, although a case in a nine-month old child has been reported. The condition occurs with equal frequency in men and women. Prior to onset, many patients have no history of diabetes mellitus. Moreover those with diabetes usually have been well controlled with diet or hypoglycemic agents. Although symptoms usually develop over a few days to a week unless an acute precipitating event is the cause, HHNK has occurred within several hours following peritoneal dialysis or major surgery. Symptoms reflect the osmotic diuresis and include polyuria, polydipsia, and occasionally polyphagia. Patients with HHNK generally have a longer history than do patients with diabetic ketoacidosis. Neurologic abnormalities are common. Unlike uncomplicated diabetic ketoacidosis, seizures are frequent in HHNK and occur in approximately 15 percent of patients. Focal signs characteristic of thromboembolic cerebral infarction are common as part of the initial presentation and frequently resolve with successful therapy. Indeed in many cases the admitting diagnosis is "cerebrovascular accident," which results in delay of the correct diagnosis and management of HHNK. Consequently, any comatose patient should have a screening test for glucose in blood and in urine so that delay in the diagnosis of HHNK is prevented. Not all patients with HHNK are comatose, half are either obtunded or stuporous, while a small percentage are alert.

CLINICAL FEATURES OF HHNK
- Average age is approximately 60 years old
- Equal frequency in men and women
- Majority of patients have no history or mild adult-onset diabetes mellitus
- Majority of patients have intercurrent illness
- Many patients have been on diabetogenic drugs
- Symptoms of polyuria, polydipsia, and polyphagia reflect osmotic diuresis
- Physical examination shows evidence of marked volume depletion and mental obtundation

---

Physical examination usually reveals extensive evidence of extracellular fluid volume depletion. Relative or absolute hypotension and tachycardia are present in the majority of patients. Skin turgor is usually poor, but the value of this sign is difficult to assess as most patients are elderly. Many individuals also have a precipitating illness such as gastroenteritis or myocardial infarction. In addition, the use of certain drugs (e.g., thiazide diuretics, diphenylhydantoin and glucocorticoid steroids) has been associated with the onset of HHNK. Hospital procedures such as peritoneal or hemodialysis, hyperalimentation, and the use of mannitol have also produced HHNK.

Laboratory Examination

The diagnosis of HHNK is easily made once the syndrome is considered. No rigid criteria have been set but a laboratory diagnosis may be defined as:

1. Glycosuria of 3+ or 4+ without ketonuria
2. Extreme hyperglycemia usually greater than 600 mg/100 ml.

INTERCURRENT ILLNESSES ASSOCIATED WITH HHNK

Infection particularly pneumonia
Cardiovascular
- Myocardial infarction
- Cerebrovascular accident
- Gastrointestinal bleeding

Miscellaneous
- Pancreatitis
- Excessive carbohydrate intake
- Surgery
- Dialysis

DRUGS ASSOCIATED WITH HHNK

- Diuretics (particularly thiazides, chlorthalidone, furosemide)
- Glucocorticoid steroids
- Propranolol
- Immunosuppressive agents
- Dilantin® (phenytoin)
- Diazoxide

---

3. Negative or minimally positive nitroprusside test (Acetest) (i.e., no greater than 2 + reaction when plasma is diluted 1:1 with water)
4. Serum osmolality greater than 350 mOsm/kg.

In the absence of an osmometer the approximate plasma osmolality may be calculated by using the formula:

$$\text{Osmolality (normal} = 285\text{--}300 \text{ mOsm)}$$

$$= 2 \,[\text{serum Na}^+] + \frac{\text{blood glucose}}{18} + \frac{\text{blood urea nitrogen (BUN)}}{2.8}$$

In any given series, the individual values for blood glucose and plasma osmolality vary widely. In one large series, the mean blood glucose was 1166 mg percent (standard deviation ± 306), and the mean plasma osmolality was 384 mOsm/kg H_2O (standard deviation ± 27).

Initial studies should include a complete blood count, electrolytes, blood urea nitrogen, creatinine, urinalysis, and arterial blood gases. Interpretation of the serum sodium must take into account the "pseudohyponatremia" induced by hyperglycemia; for every 100 mg elevation of glucose above 100, the serum sodium is reduced by 1.6 mEq/L. Knowledge of this relationship is important in determining the water deficit in such a patient. Elevated triglyceride levels might result in factitious hyponatremia. A normal or increased

---

LABORATORY FINDINGS IN HHNK

- Glucose usually greater than 600 mg/100ml
- Osmolality greater than 350 mOsm/kg
- Nitroprusside test usually negative

- Serum sodium usually normal to elevated
- Serum potassium normal to low
- BUN and creatinine and BUN/creatinine usually elevated

---

plasma osmolality coupled with a low serum sodium suggests this possibility. Many of the initial studies reflect marked intravascular dehydration. The hemoglobin and hematocrit are commonly elevated and return to normal with adequate fluid replacement. The blood urea nitrogen and creatinine are characteristically elevated as in the BUN/creatinine ratio (normally 10 to 1). With adequate treatment the BUN and creatinine will return toward normal. Many patients, even after successful therapy will have residual impairment of kidney function. Patients with HHNK have a total body depletion of potassium that is secondary to the osmotic losses in the urine and gastrointestinal tract. Unlike patients with diabetic ketoacidosis, patients with HHNK are uncommonly hyperkalemic. In one series, approximately 12 percent of patients with HHNK had hyperkalemia initially whereas almost 30 percent had initial potassium levels below 4.0 mEq/liter. In a series of patients studied by Arieff and Carroll, the mean initial values for BUN, creatinine, serum sodium, and potassium were 95 mg percent, 5.6 mg percent, 144 mEq/liter, and 5.0 mEq/liter respectively. The "normal" serum sodium, in spite of extreme hyperglycemia, reflects the tremendous loss of body water which occurs in patients with HHNK. Metabolic acidosis is not infrequent in this syndrome and as defined by a serum bicarbonate level of less than 21 mEq/liter or an arterial pH of 7.35 or less, occurs in 40 to 60 percent of the patients. Slight lactate elevations are frequent but do not account for the majority of cases of metabolic acidosis. Renal failure accounted for several. The cause for the metabolic acidosis is unkown in the majority of cases in HHNK, and in most patients it is probably multifactorial. A baseline electrocardiogram should always be obtained to identify a painless myocardial infarction. Appropriate bacterial stains and cultures should be done to rule out an infection.

MANAGEMENT

Supportive

The correction of HHNK encompasses four areas:

1. Replacement of fluid and electrolyte deficits

2. Normalization of the intermediary metabolism
3. Avoidance of complications
4. Diagnosis and treatment of the precipitating event.

All patients should have a complete and up-to-date flow sheet (Figure 3–2), which will eliminate uncertainty about previous therapy and will indicate how the patient responds to various treatment modalities. If possible, central venous pressure lines and urinary catheters should be avoided to minimize the risk of a superimposed infection. If necessary, however, a Swan-Ganz catheter is preferred to a central venous pressure line. Gastric aspiration is useful for persistent vomiting or gastric atony. If the patient is unconscious, a cuffed endotracheal tube will help avoid aspiration pneumonia.

Fluid and Electrolyte Therapy

Fluid therapy in patients with HHNK is controversial. Most authors recommend normal saline while others prefer replacement with ½ normal saline providing the patient is not clinically hypotensive or oliguric. Initial therapy is best determined by the clinical presentation of the individual patient. Regardless of the treatment chosen, careful monitoring is required to determine progress and changes in fluid replacement. Total body water loss in patients with HHNK has been estimated to average 24 percent with approximately 50 mEq/liter of sodium and potassium lost from osmotic diuresis. These losses reflect an average 8 mEq/kg and 6 mEq/kg, respectively. Thus, most patients who presented with HHNK have marked clinical evidence of sodium depletion (relative or absolute hypotension, tachycardia, oliguria, and poor skin turgor), and require rapid correction of the sodium deficit with normal saline. Each patient is an individual and the amount of normal saline required will differ. Most individuals with HHNK are elderly; as a result, sodium overload must be carefully avoided. Those patients who upon initial presentation do not have evidence of sodium depletion, may be treated with ½ normal saline. If this is done, careful and continuous monitoring of intravascular volume is necessary. Replacement with hypotonic fluids, along with simultaneous lowering of the plasma glucose by insulin, may induce hypotension and oliguria due to the movement of water from the extracellular to the intracellular space. Replacement of sodium deficit with normal saline results in a slower drop in the plasma osmolality. The average loss of water is approximately 75–100 ml/kg of body weight. The free water deficit may be calculated by the following formula:

$$H_2O \text{ deficit} = 0.6 \times BW_{kg} \left(1 - \frac{140}{[Na_{obs}]}\right)$$

Time	CLINICAL PARAMETERS				LABORATORY PARAMETERS					TREATMENT PARAMETERS	
	Blood Pressure	Pulse	Urine Output	Physical Exam	Blood				Urine	Fluids	Insulin
					Na^+ / Cl^-	K^+ / CO_2^-	pH / HCO_3^-	BUN / Glucose	Glucose / Ketones	Type / Volume	Type/Dose/Route

Figure 3–2.   Sample flow sheet for Hyperosmolar Hyperglycemic Nonketoic Coma.

Although several assumptions are made in this formula, it is adequate for the initiation of treatment. It is important to realize that the above formula does not take into account the ongoing urinary and non-urinary losses of fluid and electrolytes. Thus, replacement of free water must accommodate losses that have already taken place. Generally, replacement of the water deficit is accomplished by $D_5\frac{1}{2}$ normal saline or 5 percent dextrose as the plasma glucose approaches 250 mg percent. As the patient becomes more alert, water may be taken by mouth. Too rapid correction of the water deficit may result in water intoxication with cerebral edema (see complications on page 45). Moreover, extreme caution is advisable in those patients who present with a low plasma osmolality because removal of the osmotic effect of glucose by insulin therapy or use of hypotonic fluids may also cause water intoxication.

Total body potassium losses are probably higher in HHNK than in diabetic ketoacidosis, thus the mean initial potassium in HHNK is lower. Potassium replacement, with the chloride or phosphate salt, is generally indicated as part of initial treatment. Contraindications to early potassium replacement include electrocardiographic evidence of hyperkalemia, known hyperkalemia, and probably oliguria. Careful monitoring of the potassium levels is required as electrocardiographic evidence of hyperkalemia is nonspecific.

Normalization of the Intermediary Metabolism

There has been a shift to the use of low-dose insulin therapy in the treatment of HHNK. The main goal of insulin therapy is to return carbohydrate metabolism to normal. Hyperglycemia in HHNK reflects three conditions:

1. Underexcretion of glucose by the kidney
2. Overproduction of hepatic glucose
3. Peripheral under-utilization of glucose.

Studies have shown that circulating insulin levels of approximately 200 mU/ml are sufficient to inhibit gluconeogenesis and to produce almost maximal glucose uptake by adipose tissue and muscle. This concentration of insulin may be achieved by intramuscular or intravenous administration. An initial injection of 20 units of regular insulin followed by 10 units per hour, given into the deltoid muscle, will result in a sufficient circulating level to reverse HHNK and cause a predictable fall in plasma glucose (approximately 80–100 mg of glucose per hour assuming adequate volume repletion). Satisfactory results have been shown in the treatment of HHNK with an intravenous loading dose of 5 to 10 units of regular insulin followed by a continuous infusion of 7 to 12 units per hour. Benefits of low-dose insulin include less hypokalemia, decreased incidence of delayed hypoglycemia, and less empiric dosing. Use of subcutaneous insulin is discouraged as this route depends heavily on the adequacy of intravascular volume. If there is any doubt about the practicality of the use of continuous infusion of insulin in a given hospital, the intramuscular route is the treatment of choice. It is important to realize that no matter how the insulin is given, it is only part of the total management of the patient with HHNK.

Avoidance of Complications

Although there are many potential fatal complications of HHNK, two are of importance and deserve mention:

1. Cerebral edema
2. Vascular thrombosis.

Cerebral Edema

While cerebral edema is uncommon, it is a potentially fatal complication of HHNK. This complication should be suspected when clinical and biochemical improvement are followed by deterioration in cerebral function. Elevation of the intraocular or cerebrospinal fluid pressure (with or without papilledema) strongly suggests this possibility. Although no treatment is of proven benefit, hypotonic solutions should be stopped and hypertonic saline or mannitol begun in hope of reversing the process. In studies in animals with diabetic ketoacidosis, cerebral edema is uncommon when the plasma is not lowered rapidly to below 250 mg/100 ml.

Vascular Thrombosis

In several series of patients with HHNK, a high frequency of vascular occlusions has been noted. In many, the occlusions involve the mesenteric arteries and are overlooked clinically. Whether the occlusions precipitate the HHNK or are a complication of it (possibly secondary to extreme dehydration), is not known. Arterial thrombi may be a complication of the HHNK since they tend to become evident hours or days after the onset of the coma. Irrespective of cause or effect, vascular occlusions occur in a high frequency of patients with HHNK, and prompt recognition is extremely important.

Diagnosis and Treatment of Precipitating Event

Approximately one-half of patients with HHNK have a severe concurrent illness. In many, this is an infection with bronchopneumonia being especially common. Some will have more than one complicating illness. Moreover, patients with HHNK may develop complications during therapy. These may be related to age or to the comatose state. Since many deaths are due to complications, it is crucial that these be recognized early and treated vigorously.

REFERENCES

Arieff AL, Carroll HJ: Cerebral edema and depression of sensorium in nonketotic hyperosmolar coma. Diabetes, Vol 23, p 228, 1974

Bendezo R, Wieland RG, Furst BH: Experience with low-dose insulin infusion in diabetic ketoacidosis and diabetic hyperosmolarity. Arch Intern Med, Vol 138, p 60, 1978

Gerich JE, Martin MM, Recant L: Clinical and metabolic characteristics of hyperosmolar nonketotic coma. Diabetes, Vol 20, p 228, 1971

Hamburger S, Rush D: Hyperosmolar hyperglycemic nonketotic coma. Jour Amer Med Womens Assoc, Vol 36, p 169, 1981

McCurdy DK: Hyperosmolar hyperglycemic non-ketotic diabetic coma. Med Clin North Am, Vol 54, p 683, 1970

Tchertkoff V, Nayak SA, Kamath C, et al: Hyperosmolar non-ketotic diabetic coma; vascular complications. J Am Geriatr Soc, Vol 22, p 462, 1971

Whelton MJ, Walde D, Harvard CWH: Hyperosmolar non-ketotic diabetic coma with particular reference to vascular complications. Br Med J, Vol 1, p 85, 1971

4

ALCOHOLIC KETOACIDOSIS

INTRODUCTION

General Considerations

Most cases of alcoholic ketoacidosis are not associated with significant hyperglycemia—a factor which makes this disorder a unique metabolic condition. Its association with alcohol ingestion, first described by Dillon and Associates in 1940, has been recognized more often in recent years. Approximately 20 percent of all ketoacidotic episodes are believed to be due to the ingestion of alcohol.

Alcoholic ketoacidosis is a common medical emergency. Prompt diagnosis requires several key laboratory investigations in a patient who presents with the clinical signs and symptoms of this disorder.

Pathogenesis

Some cases of alcoholic ketoacidosis are associated with hypoglycemia. Insulin levels in alcoholic ketoacidosis are relatively low while circulating concentrations of the anti-insulin hormones, cortisol and growth hormone, are elevated. This condition favors the mobilization of free fatty acids from adipose tissue. Free fatty acids are extremely high in alcoholic ketoacidosis and well above those levels associated with prolonged fasting in normal subjects.

Alcohol probably does not contribute directly to lipolysis. During ethanol ingestion, hepatic oxidation of free fatty acids to ketones is suppressed; thus, patients with "impending" alcoholic ketoacidosis are protected to some degree by ethanol's reduction of ketone formation. In addition, acetate, a metabolite of ethanol, inhibits lipolysis. When the blood ethanol concentration is reduced, ketogenesis becomes more active and the hydrogen-ion donating ketone bodies, beta-hydroxybutyrate and acetoacetate, are produced. In addition, a neutral ketone body, acetone, is formed. Several other organic acids have been found to be elevated in alcoholic ketoacidosis, particularly the acidic catabolites of tyrosine and other amino acids. Lastly, the peripheral utilization of ketone bodies has been found to be insulin dependent.

Since insulin levels are relatively low in patients with alcoholic ketoacidosis, the production of the ketoacidosis may be attributed to overproduction and underutilization of beta-hydroxybutyrate and acetoacetate. In addition, the intravascular volume depletion associated with alcoholic ketoacidosis reduces the urinary excretion of these ketones. Another important effect of active ethanol ingestion is suppression of gluconeogenesis and reduction of hepatic glycogen stores. Food consumption is markedly decreased in most individuals with alcoholic ketoacidosis and their ability to manufacture glucose is impaired. When these two facts are combined, it is not surprising that the majority of patients with alcoholic ketoacidosis are not markedly hyperglycemic. In fact, hypoglycemia is not uncommon.

DIAGNOSIS

Clinical Presentation

The usual history of alcoholic ketoacidosis is characterized by heavy ethanol consumption several days prior to presentation. Anorexia, nausea, vomiting, and abdominal discomfort force the patient to discontinue drinking or reduce his ethanol intake. Food intake is minimal in most cases.

Originally thought to occur mainly in women, recent series have shown a more equal sex frequency. Any age may be affected. Although generally defined as a syndrome occurring in non-diabetic patients, diabetes mellitus does not protect an individual from alcoholic ketoacidosis. Physical examination reveals no specific findings, but many individuals will have the stigmata of alcoholic-induced chronic liver disease. Vital signs are nonspecific, but hypothermia should suggest simultaneous hypoglycemia. Diaphoresis is particularly common in patients with alcoholic ketoacidosis and hypoglycemia. Tests for adequacy of intravascular volume, such as neck vein distention and orthostatic blood pressure and pulse changes, will frequently uncover a significant depletion. Abdominal examination may suggest pancreatitis or acute alcoholic liver disease. However, in many instances these conditions are not present. Many individuals will have some component of alcoholic withdrawal such as hallucinations or seizures. Unless hypoglycemia or another abnormality is present, the majority of patients are conscious.

TABLE 4–1. CLINICAL CHARACTERISTICS OF ALCOHOLIC KETOACIDOSIS

Symptoms	*Signs*
• Prolonged heavy ethanol intake	• Intravascular volume depletion
• Recent decrease in food and ethanol intake	• Confusion, disorientation or coma particularly if hypoglycemia is present
• Anorexia, nausea, vomiting, abdominal distress	• Signs of intercurrent illness
• Symptoms of alcohol withdrawal	• Stigmata of liver disease
• Symptoms of intercurrent illness	

Laboratory Examination

There are no laboratory findings specific for alcoholic ketoacidosis. Laboratory tests may be divided into those of high priority in the diagnosis and management of alcoholic ketoacidosis and low priority.

High Priority Tests

High priority tests include:

- Nitroprusside reaction
- Electrolytes
- Arterial blood gases
- Glucose
- Ethanol level

Nitroprusside (Acetest) Reaction. In alcoholic ketoacidosis, the nitroprusside reaction generally indicates a modereate or large amount of ketonemia or ketonuria. In a significant minority of patients, however, the reaction may be weakly positive or negative even though ketoacidosis is pronounced. The nitroprusside reaction is sensitive to acetoacetate, less sensitive to acetone, and does not react with beta-hydroxybutyrate. Thus, patients in ketoacidosis with an elevated beta-hydroxybutyrate to acetoacetate ratio may have a weak nitroprusside reaction. In diabetic ketoacidosis, this ratio is approximately 3:1, whereas in one series of patients with alcoholic ketoacidosis the ratio was over 7:1, indicating a marked preponderance of beta-hydroxyrate production. Why beta-hydroxybutyrate production predominates over acetoacetate is unknown, but it is not likely due to simultaneous lactic acidosis. Whatever the explanation, the clinical correlation is clear: a patient may have pronounced alcoholic ketoacidosis (or diabetic ketoacidosis) and simultaneously have a weakly positive or negative nitroprusside

TABLE 4–2.   LABORATORY CHARACTERISTICS OF ALCOHOLIC KETOACIDOSIS

High Priority	Low Priority
• Nitroprusside (Acetest) reaction usually positive • Increased anion-gap metabolic acidosis • Plasma glucose usually normal or slightly high; may be low • Frequent mixed acid-base disturbances • Ethanol levels low or absent	• Liver function tests frequently abnormal • Pancreatic function tests frequently abnormal

reaction. As is the case with diabetic ketoacidosis, the nitroprusside may worsen during the recovery phase of individuals with alcoholic ketoacidosis.

Electrolytes.   Alcoholic ketoacidosis is one form of a high anion-gap metabolic acidosis. In several studies, the anion-gap in alcoholic ketoacidosis is approximately 25 mEq/L.

$$\text{Anion Gap} = (Na^+) - (Cl^- + HCO_3^-) = 12 \text{ mEq/L} \pm 2$$

The increased anion gap is usually explained by the beta-hyroxybutyrate and acetoacetate concentrations. Occasionally, simultaneous lactic acidosis and alcoholic ketoacidosis will occur, although most patients with alcoholic ketoacidosis have a lactate level that is normal or slightly elevated. Many times the only clue to mild alcoholic ketoacidosis will be an elevated anion gap. This abnormality is seen frequently in nearly asymptomatic alcoholic patients. The serum sodium concentrations is normal in most cases. Serum potassium levels are frequently low due to vomiting.

Arterial blood gases.   Although this syndrome is titled alcoholic ketoacidosis, many individuals will have a normal or alkalemic arterial pH. Metabolic and/or respiratory components may contribute to this. Metabolic alkalosis is often precipitated by severe vomiting. The respiratory alkalosis is frequently caused by liver disease, alcohol withdrawal, or infection, particularly pneumonia. The most frequent acid-base disturbance is a mixed metabolic acidosis and respiratory alkalosis. However, a triple acid-base abnormality with metabolic acidosis, metabolic alkalosis, and respiratory alkalosis, is not infrequent.

Glucose.   In most patients with alcoholic ketoacidosis, the plasma glucose is normal or slightly elevated. In one series the mean plasma glucose concentration was 143 mg/100 ml with a range of 75 to 275 mg/100ml. Hypoglycemia is not uncommon. Several patients with alcoholic ketoacidosis have presented with hypoglycemic coma (serum glucose range 19 to 27 mg/dl). The pathogenesis of this hypoglycemia is probably a combination of decreased carbohydrate intake and impaired gluconeogenesis.

Ethanol level.   Since most patients have abstained or lessened their ethanol intake prior to admission, ethanol is often absent or minimally present in the blood. If the ethanol concentration is significantly elevated, lactic acidosis should be suspected as a component of the metabolic acidosis.

Low Priority Tests

Most patients with alcoholic ketoacidosis will have nonspecific liver function abnormalities indicating either the acute or chronic effects of ethanol. Patients frequently will have a leukocytosis secondary to stress, infection, or inflammatory illness such as pancreatitis or alcoholic hepatitis. Anemia is frequent. The BUN may be elevated secondary to prerenal azotemia or low reflecting starvation and/or impaired liver function. Pancreatic function tests such as amylase or lipase may be elevated, but such findings do not automatically mean pancreatitis is present. Amylase is frequently elevated in intoxicated individuals and in many instances the amylase is salivary in origin.

MANAGEMENT

The treatment of alcoholic ketoacidosis is straightforward. Initial therapy consists of repletion of the intravascular volume depletion with normal saline and glucose administration for alleviation of the ketoacidosis. Saline administration without glucose may prolong the recovery time. Most individuals will correct the ketoacidosis in 12 to 18 hours; the majority of patients with uncomplicated alcoholic ketoacidosis will recover and have normal blood values within that same period. Alkali therapy is generally not needed nor is it indicated unless the arterial pH is approximately 7.10 or lower.

Insulin is rarely indicated although alcoholic ketoacidosis may occur in patients with diabetes mellitus. In these patients, glucose administration may cause an elevated plasma glucose at which time the judicious use of insulin is appropriate. Serum phosphorous levels rapidly drop during treatment. Although there are no controlled studies in regard to phosphate therapy in alcoholic ketoacidosis, serum phosphorous should not be allowed to drop below 1 mEq/dl as this level has been associated with hematologic, neurologic, and myocardial abnormalities. Any intercurrent illness must be vigorously treated since the morbidity and mortality of alcoholic ketoacidosis primarily reflects the associated illness rather than the acid-base disturbance.

REFERENCES

Cooperman MT, David HF, Spark R et al: Clinical studies of alcoholic ketoacidosis. Diabetes, Vol 23, p 433, 1974

Fulop M, Hoberman HD: Alcoholic ketosis. Diabetes, Vol 24, p 785, 1975

Hamburger S, Soloff A: Alcoholic Ketoacidosis—A review of 30 cases. Jour Amer Med Womens Assoc, Vol 37, p 106, 1982

Jenkins W, Echkel RE, Craig W: Alcoholic ketoacidosis. JAMA, Vol 217, p 177, 1971

Levy LJ, Duga J, Girgis M et al: Ketoacidosis associated with alcoholism in nondiabetic subjects. Ann Intern Med, Vol 78, p 213, 1973

5

MYXEDEMA COMA

INTRODUCTION

General Considerations

The state of profoundly reduced metabolism due to thyroid deficiency is associated with a high mortality rate and is a medical emergency. Hypothyroidism is highly variable in its clinical presentation, and, not uncommonly, symptoms may be so mild that patients are normally active. Myxedema coma, the most serious manifestation of hypothyroidism, has a mortality rate that approaches 50 percent, despite institution of appropriate therapy. Intercurrent illness accounts for much of this poor prognosis, and most cases with significant morbidity and mortality occur in the debilitated elderly patient who is oversedated and exposed to cold. Frequently, medical personnel may fail to recognize the steady deterioration of a patient in whom thyroid replacement has been suspended. Finally, prolonged and unexplained unconsciousness after general anesthesia may be the first indication of severe thyroid deficiency in an elderly patient.

Etiology

Myxedema coma may be primary from thyroid disease, secondary from pituitary disease, or tertiary from disorders of the hypothalamus (Table 5–1). Most cases of myxedema coma occur in patients with either longstanding autoimmune disease of the thyroid or in patients rendered hypothyroid by surgical or radioiodine therapy for Graves' disease. Approxiately 4 percent of patients with hypothyroidism will have pituitary insufficiency as the cause of their hormone deficiency. Recognition of secondary or tertiary

TABLE 5–1.   ETIOLOGY OF HYPOTHYROIDISM

Thyroid Insufficiency (Primary)	Pituitary or Hypothalamic Insufficiency (Secondary or Tertiary)
Idiopathic	Tumors
Autoimmune (Hashimoto's thyroiditis)	Infiltrative Disease (Sarcoidosis)
Radioactive Iodine Therapy of Graves' Disease	
Surgical Therapy of Graves' Disease	
Congenital Enzymatic Defect in Thyroid Hormone Biosynthesis	

hypothyroidism may play a crucial role in the management of myxedema coma. Intrinsic thyroid disease includes destruction of the gland from an autoimmune process (Hashimoto's thyroiditis), an inherited enzymatic defect in hormone biosynthesis, administration of goitrogenic drugs, or administration of iodide to an individual with a defect in organic binding of iodide. The most common causes of hypothyroidism are autoimmune destruction of the gland or radioactive therapy for Graves' disease.

CHARACTERISTICS OF MXYEDEMA COMA
- Majority of patients are women
- Majority of patients are elderly
- Majority of cases occur in winter months
- Majority of cases occur after hospitalization
- Majority of cases are associated with stressful events or intercurrent illness

---

Patients with myxedema coma are usually elderly females who have a longstanding history of hypothyroidism. The condition is more frequent in winter months with the majority of cases being associated with a stressful event or intercurrent illness, especially infection. In one review, almost 80 percent of the patients were female with half between the age of 61 and 70 years, and over 90 percent occurred in the winter months. Of note is that many cases of myxedema coma occur in patients hospitalized for other conditions. Use of certain drugs such as general anesthetics, phenothiazines, narcotics, and tranquilizers have been implicated in the production of myxedema coma in such patients. Excessive intake of free water resulting in hyponatremia may also play a role in the onset of the coma.

COMMON INTERCURRENT ILLNESSES IN MYXEDEMA COMA

- Infection
- Anemia
- Heart Failure
- Ascites
- Pleural and Pericardial Effusions

- Seizures
- Aspriation
- Inappropriate Drug Therapy (Dosage or Frequency)

DIAGNOSIS

Clinical Presentation

Myxedema coma is a systemic disorder. In many patients, symptoms of hypothyroidism are present for several years and are vague in onset. Earliest complaints usually include fatigue, weakness, muscle cramps, and intolerance to cold. Paresthesias, weight gain, menstrual disturbances, constipation, hoarseness, hearing disturbances, and personality changes are also clinical aspects of fully developed hypothyroidism. These symptoms with a family history of previous thyroid disease, or use of radioactive iodide for hyperthyroidism, strongly suggest the diagnosis. It is not uncommon to obtain a history of discontinuation of thyroid hormone therapy. Neurologic symptoms are common in myxedema coma; 25 to 50 percent of patients will develop grand mal seizures. Patients may even have, paradoxically, frank psychotic symptoms termed "myxedema madness."

With respect to the physical examination, hypothermia is frequent as is a systolic blood pressure of less than 100 mm Hg.

TABLE 5–2.   CLINICAL SYMPTOMS AND SIGNS OF HYPOTHYROIDISM

Symptoms	Signs
Cold intolerance	Sparse body hair
Fatigue	Puffy eyelids
Weakness	Dry skin
Weight gain	Yellow tinge to skin
Constipation	Pallor
Hoarseness	Large tongue
Muscle cramps	Delayed deep tendon reflex

Bradycardia is common. The patient is usually an elderly obese female with yellowish dry skin and hyperkeratosis around the elbow and knees. Ecchymoses may be secondary to diminished platelet count and increased capillary fragility. An enlarged tongue, puffy eyes, and scant body hair, particularly of the scalp and eyelids, are common. Thyromegaly is uncommon but a surgical scar on the neck is frequent. The thorax may reveal an underlying pneumonitis or pleural effusion. Cardiomegaly is frequent and is secondary to a pericardial effusion in approximately one-third of patients. Abdominal distention caused by ascites, paralytic ileus, or urinary retention is not uncommon. Fecal impaction is frequent. Most patients are comatose and deep tendon reflexes are markedly delayed. Differentiation of primary versus secondary or tertiary hypothyroidism is clinically difficult. Clues to this distinction are listed in Table 5–3.

TABLE 5–3.   DIFFERENTIAL CLUES OF PRIMARY VERSUS SECONDARY OR TERTIARY HYPOTHYROIDISM

Primary (Thyroid Disease)	*Secondary, (Pituitary) or Tertiary (Hypothalamic Disease)*
More Common	Symptoms of increased
History of thyroid operation	intracranial pressure
Family history of thyroid	(headache, nausea, vomiting)
disease	Visual field defects
No evidence of other hormone	Evidence of other hormone
deficiencies	deficiencies
Surgical scar on neck	Sella turcia abnormal
Sella turcia normal	Serum TSH normal or low
Thyroid antibodies positive in	
autoimmune thyroiditis	
Serum TSH increased	

Although few patients with hypothyroidism develop myxedema coma, all patients with this condition are hypothyroid. Myxedema coma does not occur without a relative or absolute deficiency of thyroid hormone though there has been a recent case report of a patient in whom the serum thyroxine level was normal. Whether or not thyroid hormone deficiency alone may result in myxedema coma has been debated. Although this has been suggested, most patients also experience a stressful event or intercurrent illness concurrent with the onset of myxedema coma. The following pathophysiological derangements are commonly seen:

- Hypothermia
- CO_2 narcosis
- Hyponatremia

- Hypoglycemia
- Hypotension
- Intercurrent illness

Hypothermia

Hypothermia is found in approximately 80 percent of fully developed cases of myxedema coma. It is probably the result of a decrease in the basal metabolic rate and production of thermal energy. It is so frequent that a normal temperature should suggest a complicating infectious process.

CO_2 Narcosis

The importance of CO_2 retention in the pathogenesis of myxedema coma was described in 1960. In a group of 26 patients with hypothyroidism, Wilson and Bedell found reductions in maximum voluntary ventilation, carbon monoxide diffusing capacity, and vetilatory responses to breathing carbon dioxide. In addition, the obese members of this group had small vital capacities and abnormally low maximal air-flow rates. Varying degrees of hypercapnia were found. However, some of the patients' pulmonary function studies had returned to normal after thyroid hormone replacement. The cause of the pulmonary disturbance in myxedema coma is multifactorial. It has been shown that the patency of the airway may be negatively affected by extreme swelling of the tongue causing respiratory embarrassment. Myxedematous infiltration of the respiratory muscles with a resultant restrictive pattern of pulmonary function is thought to be contributory to the hypoxemia and hypercapnia. Obesity is known to worsen this type of respiratory problem. Also, the interaction of hypothyroidism and low pulmonary surfactant levels might play a causal role in pulmonary dysfunction. Abnormal response to carbon dioxide inhalation indicates an abnormality in central respiratory regulation in myxedema coma. Lastly, the effect of pleural effusions, ascites, paralytic ileus, and intercurrent pulmonary infection may contribute to the dysfunction seen in myxedema coma. It is of crucial importance to realize that hypothyroid individuals are most sensitive to the respiratory depressive effects of certain drugs including the phenothiazines, narcotics, and general anesthetics. Doses should be reduced, and dosing intervals may need to be prolonged because of delayed absorption and slowed metabolism and excretion. The dose of morphine should routinely be decreased one-third to one-half the normal analgesic dose; the respiratory rate should be closely monitored. Because patients with myxedema coma may have abnormal pulmonary function, baseline arterial blood gases should be obtained at the onset of therapy; the effect of hypothermia on arterial blood gases should be taken into account. For each decrease of 1° C, arterial pH raises by .015, while PCO_2 (mmHg) decreased by 4.4

percent and PO_2 (mmHg) decreases by 7.2 percent. The percent change is in reference to the value measured at standard 37° C.

Hyponatremia

Although the total body sodium space is expanded, hyponatremia is a frequent finding in myxedema coma. Several observations have led to the conclusion that this is dilutional and secondary to the impairment of water excretion. Patients with myxedema coma have been shown to have a marked reduction in the excretion of free water loads. A phenomenon such as this might be explained by the inappropriate secretion of antidiuretic hormone. In rare instances, cortisol deficiency might contribute to the hyponatremic state. Decreased water delivery to the distal diluting segment of the nephron has also been thought to contribute to the hyponatremia. Pseudo-hyponatremia may also occur in myxedema coma secondary to the frequent elevation of the plasma triglycerides. Patients with pseudohyponatremia should have a normal plasma osmolality, however, compared to the low plasma osmolality seen in true hyponatremia. Whatever the mechanism, coma and seizures may occur secondary to a low serum sodium, especially at levels below 110–115 mEq/liter. Thyroid hormone replacement is needed for full correction of the hyponatremic state.

Hypoglycemia

Hypoglycemia is uncommon in myxedema coma unless the deficiency of thyroid hormone is secondary to a pituitary or hypothalamic defect. In this circumstance, adrenal insufficiency may coexist. Intravenous glucose solutions are indicated in the treatment of myxedema coma; however, excessive free water can worsen a preexisting hyponatremia. Caution must be used with glucose replacement in hypoglycemia.

Hypotension

Severe myxedema coma is frequently associated with marked hypotension. Most of these patients will respond to thyroid hormone therapy; others will respond to adequate volume expansion with saline-containing solutions. If still hypotensive, vasopressor therapy may be necessary. Due to their synergistic effects on the myocardium, caution must be exercised in the concomitant use of vasopressor and thyroid hormone therapy. Cardiovascular monitoring during treatment is mandatory.

Intercurrent Illness

Thyroid hormone deficiency in the absence of associated stress or intercurrent illness is an uncommon cause of myxedema coma. Most patients have an intercurrent illness with infection being the most frequent. Infection accelerates the metabolic disposal and fractional clearance of both thyroxine and triiodothyronine. During acute infections, the thyroid may have a lag period in its compensatory response to these changes in hormone levels. Thus, the increased hormone utilization and decreased hormone production incline the patient toward myxedema coma.

Laboratory Examination

The patient in whom hypothyroidism is suspected may have a number of electrolyte or radiographic abnormalities. A determination of serum electrolytes, glucose and BUN, a CBC, as well as serum thyroxine (T_4), triiodothyronine (T_3), triiodothyronine (T_3) resin uptake ratio, and thyrototropin (TSH) should be made prior to initiation of therapy. Urinary electrolytes and urinary osmolality may be helpful when hyponatremia is present, while an EKG and chest x-ray should be obtained in all suspected cases of myxedema coma.

Laboratory procedures may be divided into diagnostic and corroborative tests (Table 5–4).

Diagnostic Tests

Tests of diagnostic nature include serum thyroxine (T_4) and serum triiodothyronine (T_3) levels. The triiodothyronine (T_3) resin uptake ratio should be obtained to identify potential thyroxine-binding protein abnormalities. Thyroid antibodies should be determined. These are most prevalent and highest in Hashimoto's (autoimmune) thyroiditis. The determination of serum thyrotropin (TSH) is crucial as it will be elevated in primary hypothyroidism and inappropriately normal or low in pituitary (secondary) or hypothalamic (tertiary) hypothyroidism. Thyroid scans and uptake have no role in the diagnosis of myxedema coma.

Corroborative Tests

To assess the impact of thyroid hormone deficiency on organ system function corroborative tests are used. For example, the elec-

---

TABLE 5–4. LABORATORY TESTS IN MYXEDEMA COMA

Diagnostic Tests	Corroborative Tests
• Serum T_4, T_3 • T_3 resin uptake • Thyroid antibodies • Serum TSH	• EKG • Chest x-ray, skull films • Arterial blood gases • CBC • SGOT, CPK, LDH • Cholesterol, triglycerides • Glucose • Electrolytes • Cortisol

trocardiogram in myxedema coma classically shows sinus brady-cardia, low voltage, diffuse T-wave changes, and a prolonged Q-T interval. The chest x-ray frequently reveals cardiomegaly and a pleural or pericardial effusion. Effusions in myxedema coma usually are transudates. Anemia occurs in approximately half of the patients and is ordinarily normochromic normocytic. Occasionally, patients will have an iron deficiency anemia or be deficient in folate or B_{12}. Leucocytosis is frequently absent in spite of a stressful event or intercurrent illness. Muscle enzymes such as creatinine phosphokinase (CPK), oxaloacetic transaminase (SGOT), and lactic dehydrogenase (LDH) are frequently elevated. Isoenzymatic patterns usually reveal these enzymes to be skeletal in origin and not from myocardial muscle. Replacement with thyroid hormone rapidly restores normal enzyme levels. The cholesterol and triglyceride concentrations usually are elevated due to delayed catabolsim. Plasma glucose is normal in the majority of patients; if low, however, pituitary, hypothalmic, or primary adrenal insufficiency are suggested. Hyponatremia is a frequent finding. Occasionally, this is secondary to the elevated triglyceride concentration which is termed "factitious hyponatremia or pseudohyponatremia." Serum carotene levels, which cause the yellowing of the skin, are raised. Hypoxemia, hypercapnia, and respiratory acidosis are common findings on arterial blood gas measurement. Cerebrospinal fluid protein and pressure may be markedly elevated. Serum cortisol levels usually are normal but a normal level might be "inappropriately" low in the stressful state. The production of cortisol and its peripheral degradation are decreased in myxedema coma. Urinary metabolites of cortisol are reduced. Skull x-rays occasionally show an enlarged or eroded sella turcica.

MANAGEMENT

Treatment for myxedema coma may be divided into that of the complicating illness and that of the thyroid hormone deficiency. It is important to realize that therapy must be initiated on the basis of clinical judgement.

MAJOR COMPLICATIONS IN MYXEDEMA COMA
- Hypothermia
- Respiratory Acidosis
- Hyponatremia
- Hypoglycemia
- Hypotension

Supportive Therapy

Hypothermia

Measures must be taken to ensure heat preservation by passive methods (i.e., external rewarming with blankets). Active rewarming of hypothermic patients is potentially dangerous; peripheral vasodilation, circulation collapse, and death have occurred. Thyroid hormone replacement will slowly return the body temperature to normal.

CO_2 Narcosis

Measurement of arterial blood gases is compulsory in patients with myxedema coma. Hypoxemia, hypercapnia, and respiratory acidosis will often be found. Oxygen supplementation and assisted ventilation is frequently needed, the latter often for long periods.

Hyponatremia

Hyponatremia usually responds to thyroid hormone replacement and water restriction. Severe hyponatremia (below 110 mEq/liter), or hyponatremia associated with seizures, however, requires the judicious administration of hypertonic saline with or without furosemide therapy. Therapy may be discontinued with alleviation of hyponatremia-related symptoms or a serum of approximately 120 mEq/L. Since hypertonic saline is associated with congestive heart failure and furosemide therapy with decreased serum potassium levels, the patient and laboratory (i.e., urinary and serum electrolytes parameters) should be carefully monitored.

Hypoglycemia

Glucose in intravenous fluids is recommended. Glucocorticoids are also helpful. Hydrocortisone 300 mg per day, in a continuous intravenous drip, should be adequate. Hypothalmic-pituitary-adrenal abnormalities in myxedema coma may last several weeks after thyroid hormone therapy is begun.

Hypotension

About half of patients in myxedema coma will be relatively hypotensive or in shock. Thyroid hormone replacement generally corrects the hypotensive state and, if not, cautious volume expansion will help. Vasopressor therapy must be administered with extreme caution since patients with myxedema coma are relatively unresponsive to such agents until adequate circulating levels of thyroid hormone are available. Simultaneous administration of pressor agents and thyroid hormone has been associated with myocardial irritability, and, as a result, cardiac monitoring is necessary.

Intercurrent Illness

Since most of the morbidity and mortality in myxedema coma is associated with the intercurrent illness and not thyroid hormone

---

TABLE 5–5.   TREATMENT OF COMPLICATING ILLNESSES OF MYXEDEMA COMA

Intercurrent Illness
1. Search vigorously for a clinically suppressed infection realizing that a normal temperature in myxedema coma is inappropriately high.
2. Carefully search for other intercurrent illness associated with myxedema coma (see page 55)

Hypothermia
1. Avoid external heat sources
2. Cover with blankets

Respiratory Acidosis
1. Monitor arterial blood gases
2. Use respiratory support system if necessary

Hyponatremia
1. Free water restriction usually sufficient
2. If clinically needed, saline with the administration of furosemide

Hypoglycemia
1. Use glucose in parentally administered solutions
2. Administer hydrocortisone sodium succinate (Solu-Cortef) 300 mg/daily

Hypotension
1. Usually responds to thyroid hormone replacement
2. If needed, use vasopressor agents. Monitor cardiovascular system closely

Thyroid Hormone Replacement
1. L-Thyroxine (T_4) 400 mcg intravenously as a single dose followed by 50 to 100 mcg intravenously or 100 to 200 mcg orally each day
2. Triiodothyronine 12.5 mcg nasogastric tube every 8 hours

---

deficiency, it is critical to search for an underlying precipitating disease. Infection, particularly pulmonary, is the most common. Many signs of infection, such as fever, tachycardia, leucocytosis are masked in myxedema coma. A normal temperature is inappropriately high and should suggest an underlying infection.

Thyroid Hormone Replacement

Because of few controlled studies, the best method of thyroid replacement remains controversial. While older literature emphasizes the advantages of T_3 (Cytomel) replacement, more recent reviews direct attention to T_4 (Synthroid) replacement. Much of the latter is attributable to the newer understanding of the sources of thyroid hormones in the blood. Although T_4 is secreted by the thyroid gland, approximately 50–80 percent of T_3 comes from the peripheral monodeiodination of T_4 to T_3. In addition, views on dosing patterns and route of administration remain clouded.

Proponents of T_3 replacement therapy in myxedema coma cite its heightened metabolic activity, rapid onset of action, and short half life. T_3 activity usually begins in six hours with a serum half-life of one day. Intravenous preparations of T_3 are not available commercially so T_3 is usually given by nasogastric tube. Optimal dosage is not known; dosage ranges from 10 mcg every 12 hours to 100 mcg every six hours. A reasonable dose of T_3 is 12.5 mcg every 8 hours. T_3 therapy has been complicated by angina, myocardial infarction, and cardiac irritability especially when the agent is given intravenously.

Recent studies have advocated the use of T_4 replacment because of its smoother effect, longer activity, and because a portion is monodeiodinated to T_3 in the peripheral tissues. Studies have shown that approximately 500-700 mcg of T_4 are required to restore a patient in myxedema coma to a low-normal euthyroid state.

The preferred route of administration is intravenous since oral and intramuscular absorption is variable. 400 mcg of intravenous T_4 in a single dose followed by 50 to 100 mcg intravenously or 100 to 200 mcg orally each day seems to be an acceptable regimen. The initial dose may be decreased depending on the presence of restrictive factors such as cardiac disease. In a patient with angina or arrhythmias, the initial dose may be decreased to 300 mcg intravenously. Although not as rapid as T_3, the activity of T_4 is not unreasonably delayed and cardiac toxicity is probably less. With this regimen, TSH levels begin to fall in 24 hours and usually will return to normal in seven to ten days. T_4 levels reach the normal range in one to two days.

REFERENCES

Forester CF: Coma in myxedema. Arch Intern Med, Vol 111, No 734, 1963

Hantman D, Rossier B, Zohlman R, et al: Rapid correction of hyponatremia in the syndrome of inappropriate secretion of antidiuretic hormone: An alternative treatment to hypertonic saline. Ann Intern Med, Vol 78, No 870, 1973

Hovery DM, Goodner CJ, Nicoloff JT, et al: Treatment of myxedema coma with intravenous thyroxine. Arch Intern Med, Vol 113, No 89, 1964

McConnahey WM: Diagnosing and treating myxedema and myxedema coma. Geriatrics, Vol 4, No 61, 1978

Perlmutter M, Cohn H: Myxedema crisis of pituitary or thyroid origin.

Amer J Med, Vol 36, No 833, 1964

Ridgway EC, McCammon JA, Benotti J, et al: Acute metabolic responses in myxedema to large doses of intravenous L-thyroxine. Ann Intern Med, Vol 77, No 549, 1972

Senior RM, Birge SJ, Wessler S, et al: The recognition and management of myxedema coma. JAMA, Vol 217, No 61, 1971

Sterling FH, Richter JS, Gianpetro AM: Inappropriate antidiuretic hormone secretion and myxedema: Hazards in management. Am J Med Sci, Vol 253, No 697, 1978

Wilson WR, Bedell GM: Pulmonary abnormalities in myxedema. J Clin Invest, Vol 39, No 42, 1960

6

HYPERTHYROID CRISIS ("Thyroid Storm")

INTRODUCTION

Background

Hyperthyroid crisis is a grave medical emergency resulting from augmented thyrotoxicosis, often precipitated by intercurrent illness, general anesthesia, or surgery, especially on the thyroid gland, in an untreated or poorly controlled thyrotoxic patient. Although thyroid storm has become less frequent due to improved management of thyroid disease, the entity still represents a potentially fatal condition when it occurs. The disease is usually abrupt in onset and frequently is related to a precipitating factor (see Table 6–1). Prompt recognition and effective treatment of this disorder have been shown to decrease the mortality rate. Thyrotoxic crisis (thyroid storm) is the life-endangering exaggeration of thyrotoxicosis. Before the use of iodine and antithyroid drugs, thyrotoxic crisis was associated with a mortality rate as high as 70 percent. Recently, cases which have met strict criteria for the diagnosis of thyroid storm have shown a mortality rate of 10–15 percent. In the past, thyrotoxic crisis was most commonly associated with surgical procedures. At the present time, this emergency is more frequently observed as a complication of stress, therapy, or intercurrent medical illness.

Few, if any, cases of thyrotoxic crisis arise in a previously normal individual. Most patients in whom thyrotoxicosis crisis develops have had thyrotoxicosis due to Graves' disease for several months. Although some patients develop thyrotoxic crisis spontaneously, the majority have an intercurrent medical illness or stress (Table

TABLE 6-1.   PRECIPITATING FACTORS IN THYROTOXIC CRISIS

Medical	*Surgical*
Infection	Thyroid Surgery
Pulmonary Embolus	● Appendicitis
Ketoacidosis	● Preeclamsia with
Hypoglycemia	Forceps Delivery
Digitalis Intoxication	● Tooth Extraction
Thyroid Hormone	
Intoxication	
₁131 Therapy	
Palpation of the	
Thyroid	
in a Thyrotoxic Patient	
Vascular Accident	

6–1). With the introduction of antithyroid drugs, "surgical storm" has become a rare cause of thyrotoxic crisis. Vigorous treatment of the precipitating event is essential since frequently it aborts the storm. Mortality is often a result of intercurrent illness rather than the thyrotoxic state.

Etiology

Evidence suggesting that an abrupt increase in thyroid hormone levels might cause the thyrotoxic crisis include cases which have occurred after thyroid hormone intoxication, after palpation of the thyroid in a patient with thyrotoxicosis, during therapy of Graves' disease, and after withdrawal of antithyroid therapy. The above patients were shown to have sudden increases in circulating thyroid hormone levels. In addition, thyrotoxic crisis has been reported in a patient with uncomplicated thyrotoxicosis upon the administration of triiodothyronine. Some studies have shown a slightly higher mean level of thyroxine in patients with thyrotoxic storm as compared with those having uncomplicated thyrotoxicosis. Other studies, however, have not verified this. The ingestion of large amounts of desiccated thyroid and triiothyronine in patients with thyrotoxicosis ordinarily does not cause thyrotoxic crisis. What is of greater importance than the total circulating thyroid hormone level is the amount of free thyroid hormone. Ether anesthesia and a variety of nonthyroid surgical procedures have been shown to raise the level of free thyroxine. Studies comparing free thyroid hormone levels in patients with uncomplicated thyrotoxicosis and in patients with thyrotoxic crisis are clearly needed.

Many of the symptoms and signs of thyrotoxic crisis resemble catecholamine overactivity. However, metabolism of these substances seems unaltered although catecholamine excretion may be low in thyrotoxic crisis. Epinephrine and thyroid hormone have been shown to have an additive effect on the heart of a patient with thyrotoxicosis. Although it is not clear what role catecholamines play in thyrotoxic crisis, the use of beta-adrenergic blockers has been helpful in the treatment of the patients with both thyrotoxicosis and thyrotoxic crisis.

DIAGNOSIS

Clinical

Thyrotoxic crisis is a clinical diagnosis and has been defined as a life-endangering augmentation of the symptoms of thyrotoxicosis. Most often crisis is characterized by a rapidly developing, overwhelming exaggeration of all manifestations of hyperthyroidism, resulting in decompensation of other bodily systems. Generally accepted diagnostic criteria include:

1. A temperature higher than 100° F
2. Marked tachycardia out of proportion to the fever
3. Exaggerated manifestations of thyrotoxicosis
4. In most cases, dysfunction of the central nervous system, cardiovascular system or gastrointestinal system.

Thyrotoxic crisis rarely arises de novo, and most patients who experience crisis have had underlying Graves' Disease. Numerous conditions including ketoacidosis, thyroidal therapy, thyroid hormone intoxication, and hypoglycemia have been suspected as causes of thyrotoxic crisis, but the most common precipitating factor is infection. Thyrotoxic crisis develops rapidly, usually within 24 hours. Symptoms and signs generally are an extension of the underlying thyrotoxicosis (Table 6–2). Restlessness, nervousness, diaphoresis, and emotional lability are common. Gastrointestinal symptoms include weight loss, diarrhea, and abdominal pain. Cardiac manifestations are palpitations and signs of heart failure. Neural presentations range from the psychotic state to the rare individual who displays mental apathy and coma as thyrotoxic crisis develops. Other signs of thyrotoxic crisis include fever, occasionally as high as 106° F, marked tachycardia, thyromegaly, and hepatomegaly with jaundice. The cardiovascular, pulmonary, gastrointestinal, and central nervous system abnormalities may be so marked as to obscure the thyrotoxic state, especially in the elderly.

Laboratory Examination

There are no laboratory tests that clearly separate uncomplicated thyrotoxicosis from thyrotoxic crisis. Treatment for thyrotoxic cri-

TABLE 6–2.   SYMPTOMS AND SIGNS OF THYROTOXIC CRISIS

Symptoms	Signs	
Cardiovascular Palpitations Shortness of breath Edema	**Systemic** Fever Sweating	**Nervous System** Hyperreflexia Tremor Psychosis
Gastrointestinal Diarrhea Jaundice Weight Loss	**Cardiovascular** Tachycardia Arrhythmias Congestive heart failure	Apathy Coma **Endocrine** Thyromegaly Exophthalmus
Nervous System Weakness Apathy Psychosis	**Gastrointestinal** Hepatomegaly Jaundice	

sis should be based on clinical judgement alone. Nevertheless, a number of laboratory abnormalities are associated with thyrotoxicosis (see Table 6–3). The patient in whom thyrotoxic crisis is suspected shuld have a T_3, T_4, and FTI level drawn, in addition to electrolyte determinations and glucose level. When hypoadrenalism may co-exist, a serum cortisol level should also be drawn. A two hour elevated thyroidal uptake of radioidine is suggestive, but non-diagnostic of thyroid storm and is not necessary in the initial evaluation. Thyroid function tests are elevated in the overwhelming majority of cases of thyrotoxic crisis but are not significantly different than those of uncomplicated thyrotoxicosis. Rare cases have been described with normal thyroxine (T_4) levels. A recent study has described two patients with thyrotoxicosis without elevated triiodothyronine (T_3) levels; the normal level was attributed to severe non-thyroidal illness. Finally, an absent response to TRH is also suggestive of hyperthyroidism. The increased incidence of hyperglycemia in thyrotoxic crisis is secondary to numerous events

TABLE 6–3.   COMMON LABORATORY ABNORMALITIES IN THYROTOXIC CRISIS

Hematology	Chemistry

Anemia
Leukocytosis
  (relative
  lymphocytosis
  with neutropenia)
	Increased or decreased sodium
	Decreased potassium
	Increased calcium
	Increased glucose
	Abnormal liver function tests
	High (BUN)

including decreased insulin release, increased insulin degradation, increased glycogenolysis and rapid absorption of intestinal glucose. Hypercalcemia is relatively frequent and normally mild but occasionally requires acute management with saline and furosemide administration.

MANAGEMENT

The emergency treatment of thyrotoxic crisis has five components:

1. Identification of precipitating cause
2. Inhibition of hormonal biosynthesis
3. Blockage of hormone release
4. Antagonism of peripheral effects of thyroid hormone
5. Establishment of adequate supportive care (see Table 6–4).

Inhibition of Hormonal Biosynthesis

Although either methimazole (Tapazole®) or Propylthiouracil® (PTU) may be used for inhibition of hormonal biosynthesis, most physicians would probably choose PTU. This is due to the additional effect of PTU in inhibiting the monodeiodination of thyroxine (T_4) to triiodothyronine (T_3) in the peripheral tissues. The blood level of triiodothyronine may be reduced by as much as 50 percent one day after PTU administration. This effect on thyroxine metabolism is not shared by methimazole. The initial loading dose of PTU should be large, approximately 1000 mg. Daily doses of PTU, thereafter, should be about 600 mg until the thyrotoxicosis is controlled. Depending on the total body stores of thyroid hormone, Tapazole or PTU may take up to two months to achieve a euthyroid state. Since neither PTU or methimazole is available for parenteral use, the oral route must be used.

Blockade of Hormone Release

Sodium iodide given orally or parenterally is the treatment of choice in inhibiting hormone release. Either Lugol's solution, (6.3 mg iodine per drop) 30 drops per day orally, or sodium iodide, 1 Gm as a slow intravenous drip every 12 hours, is sufficient to produce a prompt and signficant fall in the secretion thyroxine. It must be understood that iodide therapy is only temporary treatment. It has been found that patients with a good clinical and hormonal response to iodide therapy had relapsed clinically at two weeks and biochemically at four weeks. Iodide therapy must not be given for at least one to two hours after the PTU or methimazole loading dose. If given before, adequate blockage of hormone biosynthesis might not have been achieved thus allowing the iodide

TABLE 6–4.   MANAGEMENT OF THYROTOXIC CRISIS

Diagnostic
1. Complete history and physical examination; vigorously search for precipitating cause
2. Serum T_4 and T_3 concentration; T_3 resin uptake
3. CBC with differential, electrolytes, glucose, calcium, BUN
4. Serum cortisol
5. Chest x-ray and EKG.

Therapeutic
1. **Establish supportive care**
   a. Establish patient flow chart
   b. Adequate hydration with glucose, multivitamins
   c. Treat fever with external cooling or acetaminophen
   d. Hydrocortisone, 200–300 mg bolus intravenous, then 300 mg per day as slow intravenous drip until patient stable
   e. Digitalis therapy for congestive heart failure or tachyarrhythmia.

2. **Inhibition of hormonal biosynthesis**
   a. Propylthiouracil 900–1200 mg po as loading dose, then 400–600 per day in four divided doses.

3. **Blockade of hormone release**
   a. Iodide: Lugol's solution 30 drops per day or sodium iodide 1 gm as a slow push over 30 minutes; repeat every 8–12 hours
   b. SSKI 5 drops every 4 hours.

4. **Antagonism of peripheral effect of thyroid hormones**
   a. Propranolol
      1. Contraindicated in asthma, heart block
      2. Use with great caution in patients on insulin or oral hypoglycemic agents
      3. Digitalize patient with congestive heart failure before starting propranolol
      4. *Oral dose:* 20–40 mg every 6 hours. Dose needed may be larger. Establish dosage level which clinically is effective.
      Intravenous dose: 1mg/5 min up to 10 mg total. Monitor blood pressure and EKG. Intravenous route indicated if patient is comatose, unable to take oral medications, or heart rate greater than 140/min.
   b. Reserpine or Guanethidine
      1. May be used in patients in whom propranolol is contraindicated
      2. Reserpine 1 mg to 5 mg initially IM then 0.07 to 0.03 mg per kg during first 24 hours in divided doses
      3. Guanethidine 1 to 2 mg/kg daily.

to be utilized as substrate for additional thyroxine biosynthesis. Lithium carbonate has a similar action; it also causes a reduction in the release rate of the hormone. Serum thyroxine levels fell about 30–50 percent with either iodine or lithium with stabilization of the thyroxine level at three to six days. As with iodide therapy, lithium treatment will also be associated with an "escape effect;"thus iodide and lithium should be used only for short-term rapid suppression of thyroid hormone release. With no clear advantage over iodide, and a narrow therapeutic/toxic ratio, lithium probably is recommended only for those patients with iodide allergy.

ANTAGONISM OF PERIPHERAL EFFECTS OF THYROID HORMONE

Antagonism of the peripheral effects of thyroid hormone has been achieved by anti-adrenergic drugs. Reserpine and guanethidine, both drugs with deplete catecholamines, have been used with less than ideal results. Reserpine in an initial dose of 1 to 5 mg intramuscular, and 0.07 to 0.3 mg per kilogram of body weight in the first 24 hours, has been shown to decrease the hyperthermia, hyperhidrosis, tachycardia, and psychological aberrations associated with thyrotoxic crisis within four to eight hours. Problems with reserpine, however, include slow onset of action, central nervous depression, cutaneous flush, and diarrhea. Guanethidine has been effective in doses of 50 to 150 mg but may take several days for maximum effect. In addition, orthostatic hypotension and depletion of myocardial catecholamines may be associated with serious consequences. The beta-adrenergic blocking agent, propranolol, is the drug of choice for antagonism of the peripheral effects of thyroid hormone. Clinical manifestations responding to propranolol include psychomotor signs and symptoms and catecholamine-induced cardiac manifestations. Part of the effect of propranolol may be that this drug partially inhibits the monodeiododination of thyroxine (T_4) to triiodothyroxine (T_3). Depending on the route of administration, the response to propranolol may be evident within minutes (intravenous) or within an hour (oral). The intravenous dose is 1 mg per minute up to maximum of 10 mg. This dose should last about three to four hours. Oral therapy with propranolol is geared to achieving a plasma propranolol level of 50 to 100 mg per ml at the end of a dosing interval in order to achieve adrenergic receptor inhibition. Variable plasma propranolol levels have been found in patients with thyrotoxicosis. In one group of patients, 160 mg daily of oral propranolol was frequently too low to achieve adequate blood levels. Regardless of the route, the effect of propranolol should be made by clinical judgement. Propranolol should not be used in patients with asthma or heart block and should be used with great caution in patients on insulin or oral hypoglycemic agents; the clinical manifestations of hypoglycemia may be masked by beta-adrenergic blockage. Propranolol is a myocardial depressant and should not be used in patients with congestive heart failure. This produces a dilemma in thyrotoxic crisis because congestive heart failure may be due to, or exaggerated by, the marked tachycardia that should respond to propranolol administration. Regardless of this possibility, conventional therapy with digitalis should be undertaken before the administration of propranolol. Plasmapheresis, peritoneal dialysis, and charcoal hemoperfusion have also been used to treat thyrotoxic crisis with some success.

ESTABLISHMENT OF ADEQUATE SUPPORTIVE CARE

Patients in thyrotoxic crisis are in a catabolic state. Usually, there has been marked loss of fluid and electrolytes due to a fever, vomiting, diarrhea, and sweating. Adequate hydration with proper electrolyte composition is crucial. A high-calorie, high-protein diet should be given. Multivitamins should be prescribed. Fever should be controlled with antipyretics or a cooling blanket. Aspirin should not be used since it has been shown to displace triiodothyronine from its carrier protein and increase the free level of that hormone. Glucocorticoid therapy, 300 mg initially of hydrocortisone by the intravenous route, and 100 mg every eight hours intravenously thereafter is sufficient to cover possible adrenal insufficiency. Documented adrenal insufficiency is the rate in thyrotoxic crisis but glucocorticoid turnover and degradation is accelerated. Sedation is occasionally necessary, less so now with propranolol therapy.

Thyrotoxic crisis is a "life-endangering augmentation of the symptoms of thyrotoxicosis." Prompt recognition and therapy of this illness has produced a decrease in mortality. All patients with thyrotoxicosis are at risk; this deadly illness should be promptly brought under control. No patient with thyrotoxicosis should undergo surgery until the thyrotoxicosis has been clinically and biochemically alleviated. With treatment as recommended, the mortality of this once uniformly fatal condition should be reduced to about 10 percent.

REFERENCES

Blonde L, Skelton CL: Hyperthyroidism and cardiovascular disease: Concepts and management. Cardiovascular Med, Vol 3, p 1145, 1978

Bolanos F, Olvera S, Ruiz A, et al: Thyroid crises. Rev Invest Clin, Vol 29, p 43, 1977

Mazzaferri GL, Skillman TG: Thyroid storm: A review of 22 episodes with special emphasis on the use of guanethidine. Arch Int Med, Vol 124, p 684, 1969

Roizen M, Becker C: Thyroid storm. Calif Med, Vol 115, p 5, 1971
Rubenfeld S, Silverman VE, Welch KM et al: Variable plasma propranolol levels in thyrotoxicosis. N Engl J Med, Vol 300, p 353, 1979
Urbanic RC, Mazzaferri EL: Thyrotoxic crisis and myxedema coma. Heart Lung, Vol 7, p 435, 1978

7

HYPERCALCEMIC CRISIS

INTRODUCTION

Hypercalcemia is a common clinical abnormality. In many cases, the patient is asymptomatic and the increased calcium is discovered by routine biochemical testing. In other patients, the clinical symptomatology is mild and mainly involves gastrointestinal symptoms, central nervous system abnormalities, renal stones, and systemic findings such as fatigue and weakness. In a distinct minority of patients (usually when total serum levels exceed 14 mg percent), hypercalcemia presents as a medical emergency—hypercalcemic crisis. Such individuals present with a wide variety of manifestions including anorexia, nausea, vomiting, increased urination, severe weakness, disorientation, obtundation, or coma. Physical examination usually reveals evidence of marked intravascular volume depletion, in addition to symptoms and signs referrable to the underlying etiology of the hypercalcemia. While most cases are encountered in patients with solid tumors (particularly breast, lung and kidney) or multiple myeloma, a small fraction occur in patients with primary hyperparathyroidism or with other eitologies for hypercalcemia.

The two most common eitologies of hypercalcemia in institutionalized patients are primary hyperparathyroidism, in which parathyroid hormone (PTH) is increased, and malignancy in which PTH secretion is usually suppressed. In the general population, primary hyperparathyroidism is the most common underlying cause of hypercalcemia. Other major causes that need to be considered include immobilization, secondary hyperparathyroidism, a recent calcium load, drug-induced causes (i.e., Vitamins A and D, thiazide diuretics, lithium or the mild-alkali syndrome), nonparathyroid endocrinopathies, (i.e., multiple endocrine neoplasia types 1 and 2, adrenal insufficiency, hyper or hypothyroidism, acromegaly or pheochromocytoma), sarcoidosis, hemodialysis, and bone diseases among others.

A number of pathogenic mechanisms, both humoral and non-humoral, have been proposed to explain why hypercalcemia is often found in association with known malignant disease. The simplest of these has been the increased bone resorption in patients with direct metastatic involvement of bone by tumors such as those from lung, breast, and kidney. Mobilization of calcium might be expected to occur due to the local mediators such as prostaglandin E_2, osteolytic phytosterols, and osteoclastic activating factor may be important in normal bone resorption. Those patients whose tumors appear to release substances into the blood that cause bone resorption and increase the serum calcium even when there has been no direct bone invasion is another mechanism of interest.

The hypercalcemia of malignancy has also been associated with increased concentrations of circulating parathyroid hormone (PTH). The increase in assayed PTH levels could be due to either an undetected parathyroid adenoma being present in the face of malignancy or tumor generated PTH-like substances.

A recent development in the biochemical evaluation of patients with cancer-associated hypercalcemia or hyperparathyroidism has been the quantitation of nephrogenous cyclic adenosine monophosphate (AMP). Data suggests that elevated excretion of urinary cyclic AMP could be a useful marker of humorally mediated cancer-associated hypercalcemia and that the various subtypes of cancer-associated hypercalcemia are biochemically different from primary hyperparathyroidism. The future role of this exam remains to be defined.

DIAGNOSIS

Clinical Presentation

Because the clinical signs and symptoms of hypercalcemia are non-specific, laboratory tests must be relied upon to establish the diagnosis. The most commonly seen clinical manifestations of hypercalcemia include polyuria, polydipsia, nausea, vomiting, confusion, anorexia, constipation, and muscle weakness. Progressive increase in the serum calcium may lead to coma and arrhythmias, accompanied by characteristic ECG changes of prolonged PR and shortened QT intervals, depressed T waves, and heart block.

Laboratory

Initial tests for a patient suspected of being in hypercalcemic crisis include BUN, creatinine, electrolytes, phosphate, calcium, and magnesium.

Although specific assay methods can allow for the measurement of ionized calcium (Ca^{++}), the most common laboratory measurement of calcium is that of the total serum calcium. The total serum calcium is comprised of non-diffusable protein-bound calcium (39.5 percent) and two diffusable components; ionized calcium (46.9 percent) and calcium complexes (13.6 percent). In the majority of situations, it is the Ca^{++} fraction of the total serum calcium which is most important physiologically. In the treatment of hypercalcemia, however, it is adequate to measure the total serum calcium level to gauge the therapeutic response to treatment.

In patients with various protein disorders, it is important to keep in mind that for each 1 gm per dl that albumin goes up or down, we get a likewise increase or decrease in serum calcium concentration by 0.8 mg per dl. In those with acid base disorders, the serum Ca^{++} level varies inversely by 1.68 mg per dl with each 1.0 unit of pH change.

MANAGEMENT

General Support

Patients usually present with marked intravascular volume depletion. Therapy is aimed at reestablishing and maintaining a proper volume status. Initial treatment should include rapid volume expansion with normal saline and correction of any electrolyte abnormalities, particularly potassium and magnesium. Special and immediate attention must be paid to the hypercalcemic patient who is on a digitalis preparation. Calcium and digitalis are synergistic in their effect on the myocardium; thus, any digitalis preparation may need to be temporarily reduced during correction of the hypercalcemia. The potassium concentration should be brought to high normal range. Conversely, "digitalization" may be achieved with a smaller dosage than with the same patient while normocalcemic. In addition, usage of normal saline not only will correct the

---

TREATMENT BY INCREASED RENAL EXCRETION OF CALCIUM

Administer saline solution

Administer loop diuretic

- Furosemide
- Ethacrynic acid
- Thiazides contraindicated

Hemodialysis or peritoneal dialysis

intravascular volume but will cause a significant calcuresis when sodium deficits are fully replaced. Mobilization of the patient should be achieved as quickly as possible to prevent excessive calcium release from bones into the extracellular fluid.

Increased Renal Excretion of Sodium

After replacement of the intravascular volume depletion, continued urinary excretion of calcium may be achieved with saline administration and use of the loop diuretic furosemide. Loop diuretics promote a calcuresis by decreasing renal tubular resorption of sodium and calcium. Therapy of hypercalcemia crisis with furosemide would range from administration of 40–200 mg every 2–3 hours to 100 mg every hour intravenously. Particular attention must be paid to maintaining adequate intravascular volume and normal electrolyte concentrations during furosemide therapy. Monitoring serial urinary electrolytes and replacing urine losses (including volume) with normal and/or half normal saline plus appropriate electrolytes would be adequate. This mode of therapy is relatively safe and has a quick onset of action. Major drawbacks to this technique include the close clinical monitoring required, variability of effect, and decreases in effectiveness over time. Sodium loading with furosemide therapy usually precedes or coincides with other longer acting modalities in the treatment of hypercalcemia. Sodium sulfate or sodium citrate therapy is no longer used because of significant side effects including sodium overload, hypernatremia, and potassium and magnesium depletion. In patients unable to tolerate saline/furosemide therapy because of renal failure or congestive heart failure either hemodialysis or peritoneal dialysis may be quite effective over the short term.

GENERAL SUPPORT IN HYPERCALCEMIC CRISIS
- Repletion of intravascular volume
- Correct electrolyte abnormalities
- Monitor digitalis therapy
- Increase mobilization

Decreasing Intestinal Absorption of Calcium

Decreasing intestinal absorption of calcium is beneficial in the treatment of certain illnesses associated with intestinal hyperabsorption of calcium such as sarcoidosis and vitamin D intoxication. However, it does not play a major role in the treatment of hypercalcemic crisis. In many instances, oral or parenteral corticosteroid therapy is begun early with the hope that it will contribute to lowering the calcium level in a week or two. The response of hypercalcemia associated with malignancy is variable to steroid therapy whereas hypercalcemia induced by sarcoidosis or vitamin D intoxication has a good response.

Decreasing Movement of Calcium from Bone

Inhibition of bone resorption is achieved most effectively with mithramycin. This drug is particularly useful with hypercalcemia associated with a malignancy. Significant lowering of the calcium level may take 1–3 days; thus, one must be cautious before administering a second dose before the maximum effect of the initial dose is known. The preferred dosage is 25 mcg/kg given over several hours. Mithramycin may produce profound and prolonged hypocalcemia. Additional side effects include nausea, vomiting, and bleeding associated with thrombocytopenia. Hepatic and renal dysfunction may occur.

Calcitonin is a second drug commonly used to inhibit bone resorption. Salmon calcitonin appears to be the most effective form in regard to potency and duration of action. Response to calcitonin is variable and usually of a short duration. Simultaneous corticosteroid administration may increase the duration of action. Calcitonin may be given either intravenously or intramuscularly at a dosage of 4–8 MRC units per kg every 6 to 12 hours. Serious side effects are rare; nausea and vomiting occasionally occurs.

TREATMENT BY DECREASING MOVEMENT OF
CALCIUM FROM BONE
1. Mithramycin
2. Calcitonin

Increase Movement of Calcium from Extracellular Fluid

Inorganic phosphates are the major drugs used to achieve this treatment principle. Serum calcium may drop precipitously secondary to intravenous phosphate administration. Although used frequently in the past, the introduction of newer drugs such as mithramycin and calcitonin and the vigorous administration of saline and furosemide have relegated intravenous phosphate administration to a secondary role in the treatment of hypercalcemic crisis. Intravenous phosphate should be given in a dosage not more than 50 mmoles of elemental phosphorous over 6–8 hours; only one dose should be given per 24 hours. A magnesium level should always be checked prior to phosphate administration. Serum calcium should begin to drop immediately; the maximum decrease may take several days. Side effects include:

- Hypocalcemia
- Profound hypotension (if the phosphorous is given too rapidly)
- Manifestations of metastatic calcification including pruritus and renal insufficiency.

> ### TREATMENT BY INCREASING MOVEMENT OF CALCIUM INTO BONE
> Inorganic phosphorous
> - Intravenous in emergency situations
> - Oral in prolonged therapy

Phosphorous is contraindicated with renal failure or significant hyperphosphatemia. Although of value in prolonged therapy of hypercalcemia, oral phosphorous preparations have a limited role in the acute therapy of hypercalcemia crisis. Prostaglandin synthesis inhibition such as indomethacin or aspirin have no role in acute therapy.

Treatment of the Underlying Disorder

Hypercalcemic crisis does not arise de novo but is superimposed upon an underlying disorder—in most cases a malignancy. Effective therapy of the associated illness is critical to prolonged correction of the hypercalcemia state. As most therapy will be delayed in onset, treatment of the underlying disorder does not play a major role in the acute therapy of hypercalcemic crisis.

Hypercalcemic crisis is a medical emergency which in most cases is associated with an underlying malignancy. Treatment principles include those elaborated upon in this chapter. The severity of the underlying disorder and the clinical status of the patient should determine how aggressive one will be in their therapy.

REFERENCES

Deftos LJ: Medical management of the hypercalcemia of malignancy. Ann Rev Med, Vol 25, p 323, 1974

Goldsmith RS: Treatment of hypercalcemia. Med Clin North Am, Vol 56, p 951, 1972

Schneider AB, Sherwood LM: Calcium homeostasis and pathogenesis and management of hypercalcemia disorders. Metabolism, Vol 23, p 975, 1974

Scholz DA, et al: Diagnostic considerations in hypercalcemic syndromes. Med Clin North Am, Vol 56, p 941, 1972

Singer FR, Bethune JE, Massry SG: Hypercalcemia and hypocalcemia. Clin Nephrol, Vol 7, p 154, 1977

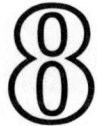

HYPOMAGNESEMIA

INTRODUCTION

Magnesium is one of the most abundant elements in the body; it is the fourth most plentiful cation and the second most abundant intracellular element. Nevertheless, the clinical relevance of magnesium has only been demonstrated in recent years. Accordingly, it is the purpose of this chapter to review the pathophysiology, clinical consequences, and treatment of hypomagnesemia, the most common abnormality in magnesium balance.

PATHOPHYSIOLOGY

The normal adult body contains approximately 20–30 gm or 2000 mEq of magnesium. Half of this amount is in the skeleton; the other half is almost equally distributed between muscle and nonmuscular soft tissue. Magnesium is located predominantly within cells. The normal serum concentration is approximately 1.5 to 2.0 mEq/L. Similar to calcium, magnesium is present in two principal forms—ionized (the main form) and protein bound which is approximately 35 percent. The average daily intake of magnesium is about 25 mEq or 300 mg, most of which comes from green vegetables, meat, grains, and seafood. An approximate intake of 0.30–0.35 mEq/kg of body weight per day is needed to maintain a normal balance. Approximately 30–60 percent of magnesium is absorbed in the small intestine; in addition, a minor percentage is retained in the large intestine. About one third of ingested magnesium is excreted in the urine; fecal excretion reflects principally unabsorbed magnesium as little is secreted into the gut. Since there is little control of intestinal absorption of magnesium, excessive dietary amounts are readily absorbed; thus, the kidney is the principal regulator of total body magnesium. Although almost 2000 mg of magnesium are filtered through the kidneys each day, only 3–5 percent of filtered magnesium is lost in the urine. This is due to an effective tubular resorption. In fact, subjects placed on a low magnesium diet will rapidly decrease their renal loss to a level that will protect effectively against hypomagnesemia.

PREVENTION OF HYPOMAGNESEMIA

In patients on prolonged intravenous therapy add 1–2 gm of magnesium sulfate (8–16 mEq magnesium) to the daily fluid requirement.

Hypomagnesemia develops from decreased intake, decreased intestinal absorption, excessive intestinal loss, and increased urinary losses (Table 8–1). The most common causes of magnesium deficiency seen in clinical practice include malabsorption, intestinal bypass surgery, diuretic therapy, and severe diarrhea. Many conditions of hypomagnesemia have multiple causes. Alcohol withdrawal is a good example; such patients have reduced their magnesium intake and have increased intestinal losses secondary to vomiting and diarrhea. In addition, secondary hyperaldosteronism, which is commonly present in chronic alcoholics, produces renal magnesium wasting. Alcohol itself may also inhibit tubular reabsorption of magnesium. Lastly, respiratory alkalosis, a common acid-base abnormality in alcohol withdrawal, produces an intra-

---

TABLE 8–1.   CAUSES OF MAGNESIUM DEPLETION

Decreased Intake
- Starvation
- Prolonged intravenous therapy

Decreased Intestinal Absorption
- Malabsorption syndromes
- Surgical resection of small intestine

Increased Intestinal Losses
- Prolonged nasogastric suction
- Laxative abuse
- Diarrhea

Increased Urinary Losses
- Diuretic therapy
- Diabetes mellitus
- Hyperparathyroidism
- Renal tubular acidosis
- Hyperaldosteronism

Transcellular Shift of Magnesium*
- Insulin therapy**
- Respiratory alkalosis

Multiple causes
- Diabetic ketoacidosis
- Alcohol withdrawal

---

*Total body magnesium content may be normal
**Particularly during therapy of diabetic ketoacidosis

cellular magnesium shift. It is important to realize that since magnesium is predominantly an intracellular cation, hypomagnesium does not necessarily mean that total body magnesium depletion is present. Nevertheless, determinations of serum magnesium remains the most practical method to detect magnesium deficiency.

DIAGNOSIS

Presentation

The predominant manifestations of hypomagnesium are neurologic and cardiac (Table 8–2). Neurologic symptoms include tremors, restlessness, fasciculations, mental disturbances, convulsions, coma, and tetany. Importantly, it is clinically impossible to distinguish tetany due to hypomagnesemia from tetany due to hypocalcemia. In fact, hypocalcemia is a common electrolyte disturbance associated with magnesium depletion. Several studies have shown that magnesium deficiency may inhibit the synthesis, secretion, and/or peripheral action of parathormone which results in a functional hypoparathyroid state and hypocalcemia. Physical examination commonly reveals positive Chvostek's and Trousseau's signs.

Cardiac manifestations include supraventricular tachycardias and ventricular arrhythmias. Whether these disturbances are related solely to magnesium depletion or to associated electrolyte abnormalities, such as hypokalemia, is unknown.

TABLE 8–2.   MANIFESTATIONS OF MAGNESIUM DEFICIENCY

Neurologic	*Cardiovascular*
• Tremors	• Supraventricular arrhythmias
• Vertigo	• Ventricular arrhythmias
• Depression	
• Irritability	
• Psychotic behavior	
• Tetany	

Laboratory

No routine laboratory finding is specific for hypomagnesemia. Other electrolyte abnormalities, particularly hypocalcemia and hypokalemia, frequently accompany hypomagnesemia. The hypokalemia may possibly be secondary to a defect in renal potassium conservation. Hyperphosphatemia occasionally is found. Electrocardiographic abnormalities present with magnesium depletion include:

- Nonspecific ST-segment depressions
- Decreased amplitude of T waves
- Prolongation of the QT interval
- Occasional shortening of the ST segment.

Other laboratory disturbances found in the magnesium deficient patient reflect the underlying disorder.

LABORATORY FINDINGS IN MAGNESIUM DEPLETION
Hypocalcemia, hypokalemia
Hypophosphatemia, occasional hyperphosphatemia
Electrocardiographic abnormalities
- Nonspecific S-T segment abnormalities
- Decreased amplitude of T waves
- Prolongation of QT segment

TREATMENT

Prevention

The approximate daily requirement of magnesium is 300–400 mg of which 30–60 percent is absorbed from the gastrointestinal tract. Thus, a patient who has no oral intake and is being maintained on intravenous fluids should receive 100–200 mg (8 to 16mEq) of magnesium daily. This amount of magnesium is present in one or two gm of magnesium sulfate.

Therapy of Magnesium Deficiency

Emergency treatment of magnesium depletion is indicated in alcoholic withdrawal seizures and ventricular arrhythmias. The former should be treated with a loading dose of 4 gm (33 mEq) of magnesium as a 10 to 20 percent solution of magnesium sulfate given over 5 to 10 minutes by either continuous intravenous infusion or intramuscular administration (see Table 8–3). Therapy then should be continued as in Table 8–4 until replacement is complete. Ventricular arrhythmias should be treated with 2 gm (16 mEq) of magnesium sulfate as a 10 to 20 percent solution over 5 to 10 minutes followed by therapy (Table 8-3) until magnesium replenishment is achieved. Intravenous magnesium sulfate should not be given as 50 percent solution. A 20 ml dose of 20 percent solution (4 gm) can be made by mixing 8 ml of 50 percent magnesium sulfate solution and 12 ml of sterile distilled water. Magnesium sulfate should not be infused more rapidly than 1 mEq/minute. Magnesium deficient patients generally require 1–2 mEq/kg for parenteral replacement. Replacement should occur over a 3 to 5 day period as

TABLE 8–3. EMERGENCY TREATMENT OF MAGNESIUM DEFICIENCY

Symptom	Treatment
Alcoholic withdrawal seizures	4 gm (33 mEq) MgSO₄* As a 10–20% solution over 5–10″ intravenously. Then treat as in Table 8–5.
Ventricular arrhythmias	2 gm (16 mEq) MgSO₄ As a 10–20% solution over 5–10″ intravenously. Then treat as in Table 8–5.

*Each magnesium sulfate molecule contains 8.1 mEq/gm.

outlined in Table 8–4 except in emergency conditions. Renal function must be ascertained prior to the initiation of magnesium therapy. Renal insufficiency does not contraindicate therapy but necessitates modification of dosage. Serum magnesium levels should be frequently monitored during therapy. A clinical clue to an elevated magnesium concentration is a decrease in deep tendon reflexes. In addition, there is no advantage to intravenous over intramuscular magnesium therapy. The intramuscular route should be utilized except in emergency situations.

TABLE 8–4. SUGGESTED DOSAGE SCHEDULE FOR TREATMENT OF MAGNESIUM DEPLETION

Route	Day	Dose
Intramuscular (50% MgSO₄ solution)	1	2 gm (16.3 mEq) every 2 hours × 3 doses then 1 gm (8.1 mEq) every 4 hours × 4 doses
	2	1 gm (8.1 mEq) every 4 hours × 6 doses
	3–5	1 gm (8.1 mEq) every 6 hours
Intravenous (≤ 20% MgSO₄ solution only)	1	6 gm (49 mEq) in 1000cc of desired IV solution to be infused over 3 hours then 5 gm (41 mEq) in each of two 1 liter solutions, to be infused over the day
	2–5	6 gm (49 mEq) distributed equally in the total fluids of the day

SUMMARY

Only recently has magnesium balance been shown to have clinical relevance. Although there are numerous causes of magnesium deficiency, clinical manifestations and laboratory findings are nonspecific, and mainly reflect neurologic and cardiac irritability. Rapid treatment is required for the emergencies of ventricular arrhythmias or the seizures of alcohol withdrawal. A slower pace is suitable for replacement therapy. Guidelines for treatment are presented.

REFERENCES

Agarwal BN, Agarwal P: Magnesium deficiency in clinical medicine—A review. Jour Amer Med Women Assoc, Vol 31, p 72, 1976

Flink EB: Therapy of magnesium deficiency. Ann NY Acad Sci, Vol 162, p 901, 1969

Geiderman JM, Goodman SL, Cohen DB, et al: Magnesium—The forgotten electrolyte. JACEP, Vol 8, p 204, 1979

Massry SG: The clinical pathophysiology of magnesium. Contr Nephrol, Vol 14, p 64, 1978

Suh SM, Csima A, Fraser D: Pathogenesis of hypocalcemia in magnesium depletion. J Clin Invest, Vol 50, p 2668, 1971

9

ACUTE ADRENAL INSUFFICIENCY

INTRODUCTION

General Considerations

Acute adrenal insufficiency (adrenal crisis) is a medical emergency. Although this disease entity is uncommon, it is associated with significant morbidity and mortality. Treatment is specific and can be life-saving. Making the diagnosis requires that the emergency physician have a high index of suspicion in the appropriate clinical setting. At present, acute adrenal insufficiency no longer occurs exclusively in patients with chronic adrenal insufficiency. With the widespread use of steroids in chemotherapeutic regimens and in collagen vascular diseases, adrenal crisis is now being recognized more frequently in patients receiving ongoing steroid therapy who have had a sudden cessation or reduction in their drug dosage.

SIGNS AND SYMPTOMS OF ACUTE ADRENAL INSUFFICIENCY
- Fever or hypothermia
- Anorexia, nausea, vomiting, abdominal pain
- Hypotension, shock
- Symptoms of precipitating illness

Etiology

Adrenal insufficiency may be caused by disease within the adrenal gland (primary), pituitary gland (secondary), or hypothalamus (tertiary). The majority of cases occur because of adrenal disease. In the past, tuberculosis and disseminated histoplasmosis were the most common causes, but recently these etiologies have been supplanted by idiopathic adrenal insufficiency, which is felt to be secondary to autoimmune destruction of the adrenal cortex. Developmental and genetic abnormalities are relatively frequent causes of adrenal insufficiency in early life. Other causes of primary adrenal insufficiency include metastatic cancer, sarcoidosis, hemorrhagic destruction of the adrenal gland (anticoagulants, shock, infection, etc.), and amyloidosis. Infiltrative diseases, cancer, and postpartum hemorrhage (Sheehan's Syndrome) are frequent causes of pituitary or hypothalamic adrenal insufficiency. Whatever the underlying disease process, the management principles for adrenal insufficiency are basically the same.

DIAGNOSIS

Clinical Features

Most cases of acute adrenal insufficiency do not arise de novo, but complicate patients with undiagnosed chronic adrenal disease. Thus, a significant percentage of patients will have an antecedent history suggestive of prolonged adrenal insufficiency including weight loss, anorexia, fatigue, dizziness, and darkening of the skin (the latter if adrenal insufficiency is primary). Moreover, many cases occur in patients known to have adrenal insufficiency but who do not recognize their need for additional steroids during times of stress. The clinical features of adrenal crisis are nonspecific and include anorexia, nausea, vomiting, diarrhea, abdominal pain, fever or hypothermia, severe weakness and hypotension. Since many individuals may have enough circulating adrenocorticosteroid to

---

TABLE 9–1.   ETIOLOGY OF ADRENAL INSUFFICIENCY

Adrenal Disease (Primary)	Autoimmune (idiopathic)
	Tuberculosis
	Metastatic cancer
	Hemorrhagic destruction
Pituitary or Hypothalamic (Secondary or Tertiary)	Tumor
	Infiltrative Diseases (Sarcoidosis)
	Postpartum hemorrhage (Sheenan's Syndrome)
Suppression of Pituitary-Adrenal Axis	Reduction or cessation of long-term steroid therapy

---

accommodate life's normal demands, acute adrenal insufficiency may occur in the face of additional stress, psychological or physiological. Thus, many patients will have symptoms and signs of a precipitating event, especially infection.

Laboratory

Although the initial laboratory abnormalities are nonspecific in acute adrenal insufficiency, the constellation of hyponatremia (seldom less than 120 mEq/L), hyperkalemia (seldom above 7.0 mEq/L), elevated BUN, and hypoglycemia in a patient who is hypotensive strongly suggests this diagnosis. The patient is frequently mildly acidemic with a plasma bicarbonate of 15 to 20 mEq/L. Although hyperkalemia is frequently encountered, many patients with acute adrenal insufficiency are normokalemic or hypokalemic secondary to decreased intake and increased gastrointestinal losses of potassium. Urinary sodium losses are inappropriately high (greater than 20 mEq/L) for the degree of intravascular volume depletion present. The white blood cell (WBC) count may be elevated (greater than 10,000 WBCs/mm³) but is frequently normal which, in the presence of stress, suggests adrenocorticosteroid insufficiency. In addition, the presence of eosinophils in the blood of a severely stressed individual should suggest a lack of adrenocorticosteroid. Hypercalcemia or hyperuricemia frequently occurs secondary to volume depletion. Electrocardiographic changes are nonspecific except for changes of hyper- or hypokalemia, and the cardiac silhouette is frequently small on chest x-ray, reflecting intravascular volume depletion.

Special Diagnostic Considerations

The most specific finding in acute adrenal insufficiency is a depressed plasma cortisol. It must be remembered that a "normal" plasma cortisol in a stressed patient is inappropriately low and is highly suggestive of adrenal insufficiency.

TABLE 9–2. LABORATORY FINDINGS IN ACUTE ADRENAL INSUFFICIENCY

Electrolytes	*Others*
• Hyponatremia • Hyperkalemia though normo- or hypokalemia frequent • Low plasma bicarbonate • High urinary sodium concentration	• High blood urea nitrogen (BUN) • Low to normal plasma glucose • Low to "inappropriately normal" plasma cortisol

The definitive diagnosis of acute adrenal insufficiency is accomplished by demonstrating a low baseline plasma cortisol with failure of the plasma cortisol level to respond to exogenous administration of ACTH. At the time of presentation to the emergency physician, the following diagnostic strategy may be employed:

1. Obtain a 10 ml blood sample for baseline plasma cortisol level
2. Administer 0.25 mg of cosyntropin (synthetic ACTH) intravenously in 1 ml of normal saline
3. Obtain a comparison plasma cortisol level 60 minutes after cosyntropin injection
4. Prior to test administer 8 mg dexamethasone intravenously to cover adrenal insufficiency.

Normal response to the cosyntropin stimulation test is an increase in the cortisol level of at least 10 µg per 100 ml, or a three-fold rise. Dexamethasone does not interfere significantly with the cortisol assay. If there is any hesitation on the part of the physician to perform a cosyntropin stimulation test during the acute phase of the patient's illness,the test should be deferred until later in the patient's course. Finally, a patient should not be committed to lifelong steroid replacement on the basis of a cosyntropin stimulation test. If the one hour test is positive (e.g., failure of cortisol to rise to 10 ug per 100 ml or achieve a three-fold rise), a prolonged ACTH (or cosyntropin) stimulation test should be done to confirm the diagnosis.

MANAGEMENT

The management of acute adrenal insufficiency encompasses four areas:

1. Fluid and electrolyte therapy
2. Hormonal replacement
3. Identification of the precipitating event
4. Patient education.

Fluid and Electrolyte Therapy

Most patients with acute adrenal insufficiency are markedly intravascular volume depleted and relatively or absolutely hypotensive. Initial fluid therapy should consist of normal saline and dextrose in amounts to prevent hypoglycemia and reverse the volume deficit. It is not uncommon to need 5 or more liters of normal saline in the first 12 to 24 hours to maintain adequate blood pressure, urine output, and replace the intravascular volume deficit. General supportive measures such as oxygen therapy may be required, and when profound hypotension is present, a central

TABLE 9–3.   TREATMENT OF ACUTE ADRENAL
INSUFFICIENCY

1. *Identify and treat precipitating event*

2. *Fluid and electrolyte therapy*
   a. **Fluid**
      Intravenous infusion of normal saline and dextrose until
      signs and symptoms of intravascular volume depletion are
      stabilized. Frequently as much as 5 liters or more are
      needed in first 24 hours. Intravenous fluids required until
      oral intake stabilized.
   b. **Potassium**
      - Hyperkalemia frequently responds to volume expansion
        and hormonal replacement. If emergent treat
        appropriately.
      - Expect potassium to drop with therapy; therefore plasma
        potassium must be monitored carefully and potassium
        given if hypokalemia occurs.

3. *Hormonal replacement*
   a. Give 200–300 mg intravenous injection of hydrocortisone
      (Solu-Cortef) immediately.
   b. Follow with 100 mg hydrocortisone intravenously every 8
      hours until stable.
   c. Give 50 mg cortisone acetate intramuscularly every 12
      hours until stable.
   d. After stabilization decrease dose of hydrocortisone 20–40%
      daily until maintenance therapy achieved.
   e. When hydrocortisone dosage is reduced below 100–150 mg
      daily fludrocortisone acetate may be needed.

4. *Education of patient*
   a. Increase (double) daily steroid dosage with minor stress
      until stress is alleviated.
   b. Wear medic-alert bracelet
   c. Educate family members about adrenal insufficiency

venous line or Swan-Ganz catheter and bladder catheterization are
recommended to monitor response to therapy.

As a rule, the acidemic state corrects with volume expansion
alone, but when plasma bicarbonate is less than 10 mEq/L, or if
blood pH is less than 7.10, therapy with sodium bicarbonate is
recommended. Hyperkalemia is quite responsive to fluid and glucocorticoid replacement (see page 92) and generally needs no therapy. Most patients with acute adrenal insufficiency are deficient in
total body potassium and with volume expansion, plasma potas-

sium concentrations will frequently become subnormal. In hypo-kalemic individuals, potassium replacement therapy is indicated early in the patient's course. Depending upon oral intake, intrave-nous fluids and electrolyte supplementation may need to be admin-istered for several days after the acute episode has subsided.

Hormonal Replacement

The diagnosis of acute adrenal insufficiency is clinical so that steroid therapy should be administered empirically in the proper setting.

Although deficiencies in *both* glucocorticoids and mineralocor-ticoids occur, initially glucorticoid replacement is the most impor-tant. Steroids with minimal mineralocorticoid activity such as methylprednisolone or dexamethasone, should not be the mainstay of treatment, although the latter may be employed to provide ste-roid coverage during the cosyntropin stimulation test (see page 90).

Initial hormonal replacement for adrenal crisis should include a 200–300 mg intravenous injection of hydrocortisone acetate (Solu-Cortef®) to elevate circulating levels immediately. This is followed by a continuous intravenous infusion of 100 mg of hydrocortisone every 8 hours. Intramuscularly administered cortisone acetate may also be given 50 mg every 12 hours to ensure a continuous source of glucocorticoid in the event the intravenous route is faulty.

After stabilization, the glucocorticoid dosage may be tapered by 20 to 40 percent daily until the maintenance dose is achieved. Steroids should be given parenterally, however, for at least 24 hours after recovery from the acute phase. Oral replacement may be started when the patient achieves a satisfactory oral intake. Although a split dosage regimen of cortisone acetate was used in the past, it is less expensive and preferrable to use prednisone, generally given in a total daily dose of 7.5 to 10 mg, which may be split 2:1 or 1:1 on a twice daily schedule. Mineralocorticoid therapy is usually not needed until the daily dose of hydrocortisone reaches 75–100 mg or its equivalent. Fludrocortisone acetate is the oral mineralocor-ticoid of choice.

Precipitating Event

Infection, viral or bacterial, is the usual identifiable cause pre-cipitating adrenal crisis. Appropriate cultures and gram stains should be obtained, but empiric antibiotic therapy is discouraged. In many cases in which no cause is found, psychological stress may be the precipitating event.

Patient Education

Once the acute phase of therapy is accomplished, patient education assumes a crucial role. Many cases of crisis are preventable. Patients should carry medical identification and be knowledgeable concerning symptoms suggestive of worsening adrenal insufficiency. Moreover, family members and friends should be aware of signs and symptoms of adrenal insufficiency. In general, minor surgery, infection, or stress is best managed by doubling the daily steroid dose for three to four days until the stressful event subsides.

REFERENCES

Angeli A, Frairia R: Simultaneous diagnosis and treatment of acute adrenocortical insufficiency. Lancet, Vol 2, p 1217, 1975

Bondy PK: The adrenal cortex. In Bondy PK, Rosenberg LE (eds): Metabolic Control and Disease, Philadelphia, Pennsylvania, W.B. Saunders Co., 1980

Dixon RB, Christy NP: On the various forms of corticosteroid withdrawal syndrome. Amer J Of Med, Vol 68, p 224, 1980

Spiegel RJ, Oliff AI, et al: Adrenal suppression after short-term corticosteroid therapy. Lancet, Vol 1, p 630,1979

Steer M, Fromm D: Recognition of adrenal insufficiency in the post-operative patient. Amer J of Surg, Vol 139, p 443, 1980

Streck WF, Lockwood DH: Pituitary adrenal recovery following short-term suppression with corticosteroids. Amer J of Med, Vol 66, p 910, 1979

10

HYPERKALEMIA

INTRODUCTION

General Considerations

Disorders involving potassium homeostasis are relatively common in the practice of medicine. Hyperkalemia, which is defined as a serum potassium exceeding 5.5 mEq/L, is a potentially life-threatening medical emergency. Early recognition is essential and can reduce cardiac morbidity and mortality. Rapid institution of therapy can return potassium levels to a safe range and can prevent serious cardiac arrythmias.

Overall understanding of the mechanisms involved is essential for appropriate diagnosis and management. Total body potassium averages between 50 mEq to 55 mEq kg of body weight. More than 95 percent of total body potassium is intracellular. The high gradient between the intracellular and extracellular potassium is maintained by an energy-dependent mechanism. The relationship between the intracellular and extracellular potassium is influenced by many factors. Insulin, and the acid-base state of body fluids, are the two more important factors in the internal regulation of potassium. The external balance of potassium, or the regulation of total body potassium, is maintained by a balance between the intake and excretion of potassium. Renal excretion contributes to more than 85 percent of the daily potassium intake. Renal excretion of potassium is altered by factors that influence the secretion of potassium in the distal nephron. The gastrointestinal tract excretes 10 to 15 percent of potassium.

Etiology

1. *Pseudohyperkalemia.* This *in vitro* phenomenon is observed in hemolyzed blood samples or with disorders associated with

TABLE 10–1.   CAUSES OF HYPERKALEMIA

Pseudohyperkalemia	Severe leukocytosis
	Severe thrombocytosis
	Hemolysis of blood sample
Increased Total Body Potassium	Excessive intake
	Renal insufficiency
	Decreased mineralocorticoid activity (adrenal insufficiency, selective hypoaldosteronism)
	Drugs
	• potassium-sparing diuretics
	• potassium-containing antibiotics
	• digitalis overdose
	• prostaglandin inhibitors
	Distal tubular defect
	• sickle cell anemia
	• postrenal transplant
	• systemic lupus erythematosus
Redistribution	Acute metabolic acidosis
	Acute respiratory acidosis
	Cationic amino acid administration
	Hyperkalemic familial periodic paralysis

extremely elevated white cell or platelet count. Prolonged use of a tourniquet may lead to elevated potassium levels in the blood sample.

2. *Redistribution induced hyperkalemia.* Hyperkalemia secondary to both acute metabolic or respiratory acidosis is due to extracellular shift of potassium. The inverse relationship between blood pH and serum potassium is influenced also by the concentration of sodium bicarbonate in the extracellular fluid, by the responsible acid (mineral versus organic acid), and by the degree of renal dysfunction.

3. Administration of cationic amino acids, such as arginine hydrochloride, may lead to hyperkalemia by an external shift of cellular potassium.

4. Hyperkalemia may be associated rarely with a form of periodic familial paralysis.

5. Drug-induced hyperkalemia is common in the presence of renal insufficiency. Potassium sparing diuretics, potassium containing non-steroidal anti-inflammatory drugs such as indomethacin, and massive overdose with digitalis may be responsible.

6. Hyperkalemia is a serious complication in acute renal failure. Life-threatening, severe hyperkalemia may occur in the oliguric patient or those with increased catabolism, such as rhabdomyolysis. Significant hyperkalemia is unusual in the steady state of chronic renal failure. Factors such as systemic acidosis, prolonged constipation, and excessive intake, however, may cause hyperkalemia in chronic renal failure.

7. Hyperkalemia seen in sickle cell anemia, renal transplantation, and systemic lupus erythematous is due to distal tubular defect in potassium secretion.

8. Hyperkalemia is a common finding in patients with generalized adrenal insufficiency as in Addison's disease. Hyperkalemia due to selective hyperaldosteronism is, however, more commonly encountered than the generalized form of adrenal insufficiency. Diabetics and those with chronic interstitial renal diseases are especially at risk.

DIAGNOSIS

Clinical Presentation

As a rule, the most prominent manifestations of hyperkalemic emergencies occur in the heart. Occasionally, however, moderate to severe elevations in serum potassium can have striking effects on the peripheral muscles. Ascending muscular weakness may occur and, in some cases, may progress to flaccid quadriplegia and respiratory paralysis. Usual cranial nerve function is preserved.

Laboratory and ECG

A variety of ECG changes are encountered when serum potassium rapidly rises above 5.5 mEq/L. The following changes are seen with increasing hyperkalemia:

- Peaked T-waves
- Shortened QT interval
- Decreased P-wave amplitude
- Widened P-wave and QRS complexes
- Absence of P-wave and sine wave
- Ventricular fibrillation and cardiac arrest.

MANAGEMENT

Management depends on the severity of hyperkalemia, rate of development, and the presence of electrocardiographic changes. Calcium salt infusion is lifesaving and recommended for severe hyperkalemia, e.g., serum potassium higher than 7.0 mEq/L, especially in the presence of significant ECG changes. Calcium administration counteracts the neuromuscular effects of hyperkalemia. The onset of action is within minutes and lasts only for 30 minutes. Solutions available for use include calcium gluconate (10 ml of 10 percent solution contains 90 mgs calcium) or calcium chloride (10 ml of 10 percent solution contains 360 mgm calcium). Administration of calcium salts should be done with continuous monitoring of ECG.

Hyperkalemia should also be treated by enhancing potassium shift into the intracellular space. Intracellular potassium shift is best achieved by intravenous infusion of either hypertonic glucose and insulin or sodium bicarbonate. Hypertonic glucose is usually administered as 500 ml of 10 percent solution with 10 units regular insulin to prevent hypoglycemia. Sodium bicarbonate administration is achieved by infusion of 44 mEq sodium bicarbonate ampules intravenously as needed. The onset of action is within 20–30 minutes and lasts only for a few hours.

Reduction in total body potassium is best achieved by increasing fecal excretion using ion exchange resin or by dialysis. Sodium polystyrene sulfonate (Kayexalate®), an ion exchange resin, removes about 1 mEq potassium for each one gram. Kayexalate is given either orally or per rectum as retention enema. Orally it is given in 15–20 gm in 30 ml of 70 percent sorbitol solution and repeated as necessary. In general, hemodialysis is more effective in removing potassium than peritoneal dialysis.

Treatment of hyperkalemia usually requires a combination of the aforementioned modalities.

Hyperkalemia due to mineralocorticoid deficiency is managed by either the administration of Florinef® 0.05 to 0.2 mgm daily, or by giving loop diuretics coupled with decreased potassium intake.

REFERENCES

Adlinger K, Samaan N: Hypokalemia and hyperkalemia. Ann Int Med, Vol 87, pp 571–573, 1977

Cohen J: Disorders of potassium balance. Hospital Practice, pp 119–128, January 1979

Nardone D: Hypokalemia and hyperkalemia. Ann Intern Med, Vol 82, pp 54–57, 1975

Patrick J: Assessment of body potassium stores. Kidney Int, Vol 11, pp 476–490, 1977

11

HYPOKALEMIA

INTRODUCTION

General Considerations

Hypokalemia may present as a life-threatening medical emergency. While gradual potassium depletion due to gastrointestinal losses, poor intake, or diuretic therapy may be asymptomatic, with moderate to severe depletion, neuromuscular symptoms including skeletal muscle weakness or paralysis may predominate. Although moderate potassium depletion rarely affects cardiac function or rhythm, severe or rapid reduction in serum potassium levels may cause cardiac arrest. Potassium deficiency enhances the cardiac toxicity of digitalis preparations. In patients who have had cardiac arrest, refractory ventricular arrhythmias should suggest the possibility of underlying potassium depletion and hypokalemia.

Hypokalemia is usually defined as serum potassium less than 3.5 mEq/L.

Etiology

1. Hypokalemia due to shift of extracellular potassium is seen in various conditions. Both metabolic and respiratory alkalosis are usually associated with low serum potassium level. Administration of glucose alone or glucose with insulin may be associated with hypokalemia. Glucose administration to diabetics with the syndrome of selective hypoaldosteronism may cause elevation of serum potassium rather than hypokalemia. Serum potassium should be monitored closely in diabetics who receive large doses of hypertonic glucose for suspected hypoglycemia.
2. Hypokalemia is a prominent feature in the familial periodic paralysis.

TABLE 11–1.   CAUSES OF HYPOKALEMIA

Internal Imbalance	*External Imbalance*
Metabolic or respiratory alkalosis	Decreased intake
Insulin or glucose administration	Increased loss
Hypokalemia familial periodic	1. Renal loss
paralysis	• Diuresis
Barium poisoning	osmotic diuresis
	diuretics
	• Acid-base disorders
	renal tubular acidosis
	metabolic alkalosis
	metabolic acidosis
	(chronic)
	• Drugs
	carbenicillin, penicillin
	licorice, carbenoxalone
	acetazolamide
	Mineralocorticoid hyperactivity
	Primary
	• primary aldosteronism
	• nonaldosterone
	mineralocorticoids
	• licorice, tobacco chewing
	• ACTH-producing tumors
	• Cushing's syndrome
	Secondary
	• Bartter's syndrome
	• edematous states
	• oral contraceptives
	• renin-producing tumors
	• renal artery stenosis
	• malignant hypertension
	Miscellaneous
	• Liddle's syndrome
	• hypercalcemia
	• magnesium deficiency
	• acute monocytic or
	myelocytic leukemia
	2. Gastrointestinal loss
	• Gastric fluid loss
	• Intestinal fluid loss
	• Villous adenoma
	• Laxative abuse
	3. Skin losses
	• Excessive sweating

3. Decreased total body potassium produced by increased renal losses of potassium is the most common cause of hypokalemia. Enhanced delivery of sodium and water to the distal nephron, induced by all diuretics including osmotic diuresis, is associated with significant hypokalemia. Potassium-sparing diuretics are the exception. Both proximal and distal renal tubular acidosis (RTA) are associated with hypokalemia. Diagnosis of RTA is suspected when hypokalemia is associated with metabolic acidosis, especially when diarrhea is excluded.

4. Drug-induced hypokalemia is seen with administration of large doses of carbenicillin or penicillin. Increased delivery of the poorly absorbable anions of these drugs to the distal nephron induces kaliuresis.

5. Ingestion of large amounts of licorice or its derivative carbenozalone, or occasionlly chewing tobacco, is associated with hypokalemia.

6. Hypokalemia is a common feature with syndromes associated with mineralocorticoid hyperactivity. Metabolic alkalosis and hypertension are usually concomitant findings. Hypertension is characteristically absent in patients with Bartter's Syndrome and those receiving diuretics.

7. Hypokalemia is occasionally seen in association with magnesium deficiency, acute monocytic or myelomonocytic leukemia and hypercalcemia.

8. Hypokalemia due to gastrointestinal losses of potassium is also common and may result from vomiting or gastric suction. The associated volume depletion, metabolic alkalosis, and secondary hyperaldosternism contribute to the renal losses of potassium.

9. Severe hypokalemia occurs with protracted diarrheal states especially with cholera and watery diarrhea hypokalemia syndrome associated with non-beta islet cell hyperplasia.

10. Villous adenomas of the colon are occasionally associated with hypokalemia. Surreptitious use of laxatives or cathartics may present the physician with diagnostic dilemma.

11. Severe sweating in a hot climate may contribute to significant losses of potassium.

DIAGNOSIS

Clinical Presentation

The diagnosis of hypokalemia can usually be suspected from the clinical history. Neuromuscular complaints, weakness, and frank paralysis are suggestive of hypokalemia. Elderly patients on potas-

TABLE 11–2.   EVALUATION OF PATIENTS WITH HYPO OR HYPERKALEMIA

1. Repeat laboratory test is mandatory to exclude error or hemolysis of blood sample.
2. Detailed medical history concerning prescribed and over-counter drugs and dietetic habits is very informative.
3. Complete physical examination to evaluate body fluid status (edema, volume depletion) and arterial blood pressure.
4. Basic laboratory evaluation to include complete blood cell count, arterial blood gasses and renal function tests.
5. Assessing the renin-aldosterone profile and adrenal functions when specifically indicated.

sium-wasting diuretics are prone to hypokalemia as are alcoholics who have decreased intake combined with diuresis secondary to decreased ADH production. Patients whose potassium deficiency is caused by surreptitious use of diuretics, laxatives, or who have psychogenic, self-induced vomiting (bulimia) will rarely volunteer an accurate history. On physical examination, patients with lowered serum potassium levels may have decreased skeletal motor power or decreased or absent deep tendon reflexes.

Electrocardiographic Manifestations of Hypokalemia

Supraventricular tachycardia and ventricular ectopic beats are relatively common with severe hypokalemia, especially in patients receiving digitalis therapy. The most frequently encountered ECG changes, however, are S-T segment depression, flattened T-waves, and appearances of a U-wave. Unexplained refractory ventricular tachycardia or fibrillation in patients with cardiac arrest may be due to hypokalemia.

MANAGEMENT

Correction of hypokalemia requires replacement of potassium deficits with potassium supplements and by identifying and correcting the underlying process responsible for hypokalemia. Serum potassium level may serve as a rough guide for estimating total body potassium deficit, especially when more accurate measurements are not available. Total body potassium deficit may range between 100–150 mEq when serum potassium is decreased by 1.0 mEq/L and between 400–600 mEq when serum potassium is decreased by 2.0 mEq/L, especially in the absence of severe acid-base disorders.

Parenteral potassium administration should be restricted to severe hypokalemia or when oral intake is not possible.

Patients with severe life-threatening hypokalemia (i.e., serum potassium less than 2.5 mEq/L who are taking a digitalis preparation) should have their serum potassium restored to normal as soon as possible. Potassium chloride infusion up to 40 mEq/hour is permissable with cardiac monitoring and frequent vital signs. Patients receiving more than 10–20 mEq/L intravenously should be monitored closely; the rate of administration and the concentration in the infusion fluid should be individualized depending on the clinical condition of the patient. Potassium chloride salt is the preferred preparation especially when metabolic alkalosis is present. When hypokalemia is associated with metabolic acidosis as in renal tubular acidosis, potassium administration should precede or accompany alkali therapy.

Potassium supplements should be used with caution in patients with decreased renal function or in diabetes.

Surgical intervention may be necessary for adrenal adenomas or renal artery stenosis.

Prostaglandin inhibitors, such as indomethacin, may be useful in the management of Bartter's Syndrome.

REFERENCES

Adlinger K, Samaan N: Hypokalemia and hyperkalemia. Ann Int Med, Vol 87, pp 571–573, 1977

Cohen J: Disorders of potassium balance. Hospital Practice, pp 119–128, January 1979

Nardone D: Hypokalemia and hyperkalemia. Ann Intern Med, Vol 82, pp 54–57, 1975

Patrick J: Assessment of body potassium stores. Kidney Int, Vol 11, pp 476–490, 1977

12

HYPONATREMIA

INTRODUCTION

Disorders involving alteration of body sodium content or concentration of sodium in body fluids are common in the practice of medicine. The clinical picture is usually nonspecific and requires collaboration with laboratory findings. Clinical assessment of extracellular fluid volume, measurement of both serum and urine sodium, and osmolality is essential for diagnosis.

The normal value for serum sodium ranges between 135–146 mEq/L. Maintenance of serum sodium within a narrow range, approximately 2 mEq/L, occurs on a daily basis. Symptoms are more common when the serum sodium is less than 130 mEq/L or greater than 150 mEq/L, especially when the changes in serum sodium are acute. In contrast, slowly progressive or chronic changes in serum sodium are more tolerable, and symptoms may not occur until the abnormality is extreme.

Determination of serum osmolality by direct measurement and by calculation is necessary for appropriate evaluation. The normal serum osmolality ranges between 286–294 mOsm/Kg of H_2O. Serum osmolality is calculated as follows:

$$\text{Serum Osmolality} = 2(Na^+) + \frac{\text{glucose (mg\%)}}{18} + \frac{\text{BUN (mg\%)}}{2.8}$$

Normal serum osmolality in a hyponatremic patient indicates either pseudohyponatremia or the presence of osmotic substances other than sodium. Variations between measured and calculated serum osmolality are indicative of osmotic substances being present other than sodium, urea, or glucose (e.g., mannitol, glycerol, methanol, or ethylene glycol).

Etiology

Pseudohyponatremia

Pseudohyponatremia exists in the presence of hyperlipidemia or extreme hyperglobulinemia (multiple myeloma, Waldenstrom's macroglobulinemia, etc.). The abnormality in such cases is related to the amount of plasma that is occupied by the lipids or the proteins. Osmolality remains normal in this setting.

Hyponatremia with Decreased Total Body Sodium

This condition is characterized by a sodium deficit that exceeds the water deficit, resulting in a low serum sodium and manifestations of contracted extracellular volume. Such manifestations include orthostatic hypotension, tachycardia, dry mucus membranes, flat neck veins, poor skin turgor, and recent weight loss. Urine sodium values can be very helpful in determining the origin of the loss. A urine sodium of less than 10 mEq/L is indicative of a non-renal source of sodium and water loss. The gastrointestinal tract is the most likely origin. However, the accumulation of fluid in a "third space" secondary to an intraabdominal process, massive burns, or severe muscle trauma must be considered. In contrast, a urine sodium of greater than 20 mEq/L, in the presence of normal renal function, suggests that the source of sodium and water loss is the kidneys. Diuretic excess, adrenal insufficiency, and salt losing nephropathies are possible etiologies.

Diuretic-Induced Hyponatremia

Diuretic-induced hyponatremia is usually associated with hypokalemia. The etiology of diuretic-induced hyponatremia includes excessive sodium and water losses, resulting in hypovolemia with secondary stimulation of antidiuretic hormone by volume receptors. This results in true and dilutional hyponatremia. The potassium deficit may contribute to the hyponatremia by an intracellular shift of sodium in exchange for potassium, since this type of hyponatremia is partially corrected by potassium administration alone.

Hyponatremia associated with an osmotic diuresis results from obligatory natriuresis by the osmotic forces, even in the presence of volume contraction. Patients with diabetic ketoacidosis, mannitol therapy, and urea diuresis may have significant losses of sodium in the urine.

Adrenal Insufficiency

The hyponatremia of adrenal insufficiency is usually associated with hyperkalemia and pre-renal azotemia. The increased renal losses of sodium and water results in hypovolemia with secondary stimulation of antidiuretic hormone. This results in a true sodium deficit and dilutional hyponatremia.

Renal Insufficiency

Hyponatremia associated with chronic renal insufficiency and extracellular volume depletion may result from salt restriction and excessive use of diuretics. Excessive losses of sodium are also common in these patients when vomiting or diarrhea is present.

The salt-losing tendency or "salt-losing nephropathy" is seen in a variety of tubulo-interstitial diseases of the kidney, even in the absence of renal insufficiency.

Hyponatremia with Increased Total Body Sodium

In this type of hyponatremia, a low serum sodium is associated with an expanded extracellular volume and frequently edema. This is seen in cirrhosis of the liver, congestive heart failure, nephrotic syndrome, and acute and chronic renal failure. Water retention exceeds sodium retention resulting in the so-called "dilutional hyponatremia." The decrease in free water clearance or water retention in these disorders is multifactorial. There is a decreased delivery of glomerular filtrate to the diluting segment of the nephron and stimulation of antidiuretic hormone by a decreased effective intravascular volume. The urine sodium is usually less than 20 mEq/L, except in patients with acute and chronic renal failure whose urine sodium values may exceed this level.

Hyponatremia with Normal Total Body Sodium

A low serum sodium associated with a clinically undetectable increase in extracellular fluid volume is the hallmark of this condition. The water retention results in "dilutional hyponatremia." Characteristically, edema is absent, and urine sodium values approximate the daily sodium intake.

Hyponatremia associated with hypothyroidism is poorly understood. Proposed mechanisms include a decrease in cardiac output with stimulation of antidiuretic hormone and abnormal urinary dilution secondary to a distal tubule defect. Hyponatremia associated with adrenal insufficiency is due to an increased sodium loss in the urine, however, the defect in water excretion may contribute to the severity of the hyponatremia. Glucocorticoids may play a part in the etiology of the low serum due to their role in the maintenance of the impermeability of the collecting duct epithelium to water.

Administration of a variety of drugs, in addition to diuretics, can cause hyponatremia. Such agents include chlorpropamide (Diabenese®), narcotics, carbamazepine (Tegretol®), barbituates, clofibrate (Atromid-S®), vincristine, nicotine, isoproterenol, and tolbutamide. The mechanism of action is frequently due to stimulation of antidiuretic hormone release. In addition, chlorpropamide enhances the action of circulating antidiuretic hormone. Aspirin and indomethacin, both prostaglandin synthetase inhibitors, have been shown to enhance the action of antidiuretic hormone. Prostaglandins normally counteract the effect of antidiuretic hormone via a negative feedback system. Acetaminophen has been shown to enhance the action of antidiuretic hormone. The mechanism remains unknown. Cyclophosphamide (Cytoxan®) can cause a defect in renal water excretion which seems to parallel excretion of an active metabolite of the drug. Lastly, oxytocin may cause hyponatremia by similation of vasopressin action.

SIADH

Hyponatremia associated with the syndrome of inappropriate antidiuretic hormone secretion, SIADH, is largely a diagnosis of exclusion. This syndrome should be considered if the following criteria are met:

1. Normal renal, adrenal, and thyroid functions
2. Absence of edema and intravascular volume deficiency
3. Urine osmolality inappropriately high compared to the low serum osmolality
4. Urine sodium values that approximate the daily sodium intake.

This syndrome has been associated with a variety of benign and malignant disorders, such as central nervous system disorders, pulmonary disease, and certain malignancies, primarily lung cancer.

DIAGNOSIS

Presentation

A detailed history and physical examination are pertinent in the evaluation of the hyponatremic patient. Special attention should be given to a history of diuretic use, vomiting, diarrhea, heart disease, renal disease, and liver disease. A careful drug history is equally important.

The physical examination should be geared to determination of the extracellular volume status of the patient. Evaluation of the neck veins, mucus membranes, skin turgor, and orthostatic blood pressure is helpful.

Signs and symptoms of hyponatremia range from lethargy and muscle cramps to multiple central system symptoms, including seizures. The severity of symptoms is dependent on the rate of development and the severity of hyponatremia. Electroencephalographic changes may also be present but are non-specific.

Laboratory

Electrolytes, BUN, and urinary electrolytes and osmolality should be drawn.

SIGNS AND SYMPTOMS OF HYPONATREMIA
(Serum Sodium < 130 mEq/L)

Thirst	Restlessness
Impaired taste sensation	Confusion
Anorexia	Delerium
Nausea/Emesis	Muscle twitching
Muscle cramps	Seizures
Abdominal cramps	Coma
Depressed sensorium	Hemiparesis ⎫
Weakness	Ataxia ⎬ Chronic
Lethargy	Babinski ⎭

MANAGEMENT

The treatment of hyponatremia is dependent upon the folowing:

1. The severity of signs and symptoms
2. The course—acute versus chronic
3. The underlying disease process.

In the presence of pronounced central nervous system manifestations (such as seizures), hypertonic saline or mannitol should be administered, regardless of the etiology of the hyponatremia. These agents are used to produce an osmotic gradient. Extreme caution is necessary to avoid fluid overload by the hypertonic saline solution, especially in cardiac patients and in the elderly.

Correction of the hyponatremic state should be gradual to avoid serious complications. Diagnosis of the underlying disease process is essential for appropriate management. Drugs known to cause hyponatremia should be discontinued and hormonal replacement considered in the thyroid or adrenal deficient patient.

In hyponatremic patients who are both salt and water depleted, replacement with isotonic saline is recommended to replace volume and sodium to a normal level. In patients with an excess of total body sodium and water, restriction of both salt and water is recommended. Sodium intake should be decreased to 2 grams/24 hours for moderate to severe sodium excess. A water restriction of 800 cc–1200 cc/24 hours is usually sufficient.

In euvolemic patients, such as those with the syndrome of inappropriate secretion of antidiuretic hormone, therapy depends on the severity and chronicity of the disease. Rapid correction is achieved by administration of a loop diuretic combined with the use of hypertonic saline. This method is effective in correcting the serum sodium to a near-normal range by inducing a diuresis with simultaneous replacement of urinary sodium and potassium. Therapy includes administration of intravenous furosemide 1 mg/kg of body weight initially, followed by subsequent doses to produce negative fluid balance and replacement of urinary sodium and potassium by 3 percent normal saline and potassium chloride. The desired negative water balance can be calculated as follows:

$$\text{Desired negative water balance (liters)} = \frac{(\text{total body solute}) \times (1 \text{ liter})}{\text{desired plasma osmolality}}$$

where, mOsm of total body solute = (total body water) × (plasma osmolality)

and, total body water = (wt. in kilograms) × (60% or 70%)

Restriction of water intake to replace insensible losses only is adequate in the milder forms.

Drug therapy is recommended when the underlying cause is uncorrectable or when the syndrome of inappropriate secretion of antidiuretic hormone is not readily reversible. Demeclocycline and lithium interfere with the peripheral action of antidiuretic hormone. Demeclocycline, in a dose of 1200 or 2400 gms/day is preferred over lithium. Side effects include a high incidence of photosensitivity and a decrease in renal function, especially in patients with liver disease. Diphenylhydantoin, through its central action on antidiuretic hormone, may prove effective in SIADH secondary to central nervous systems disorders.

REFERENCES

Berl T, Anderson RJ, McDonald KM, Schrier RW: Clinical disorders of water metabolism. Kid Int, Vol 10, pp 117–132, 1976

Earley LE, Gottschalk CW: Disorders of water metabolism. In Strauss and Well's Diseases of the Kidney. Vol II, Little, Brown & Co., Boston, Massachusetts, pp 1494, 1499, 1501, 1979

Harrington JT, Cohen JJ: Clinical disorders of urine concentration and dilution. Arch Int Med, Vol 131, pp 810–825, 1973

Levy M: The pathophysiology of sodium balance. Hospital Practice, pp 95–106, 1978

Loeb JN: The hyperosmolar state. New Eng J Med, Vol 290, pp 1184–1187, 1974

Ross EJ, Christie SBM: Hypernatremia. Medicine, Vol 48, No 6, pp 441–473, 1969

13

HYPERNATREMIA

INTRODUCTION

General Considerations

Although less common than hyponatremia, hypernatremia, which is defined as a plasma sodium concentration greater than 150 mEq per liter, can present as a medical emergency. As a rule, pathophysiologic disturbances that cause renal or gastrointestinal water losses do not result in hypernatremia unless there is a disturbance in thirst or the individual is unable to drink or obtain water. Thus, hypernatremic emergencies are most commonly seen in the very young and the very old.

In the emergency setting, the main clinical manifestations of hypernatremia are neurologic and include confusion, stupor, or coma. Occasionally, focal neurologic deficits may be present; in those patients who have undergone a profound osmotic diuresis, signs and symptoms of volume depletion may dominate the clinical picture.

Etiology

Hypernatremia with Decreased Total Body Sodium

In this condition, the water loss exceeds the sodium loss, resulting in an elevated serum sodium level and serum osmolality. Hyperosmolality of the extracellular fluid stimulates the thirst mechanism and antidiuretic hormone release. Failure to respond to thirst is common in the elderly and in patients with cerebrovascular diseases. Clinical manifestations of hypovolemia are usually prominent and associated hemoconcentration may be present, evidenced by an elevated hematocrit, total protein, serum albumin, and blood urea nitrogen. In children, metabolic acidosis is usually present, as well as hypocalcemia, which may be symptomatic. Hyperglycemia occurs in 50 percent of infants with hypernatremia. Sources of hypotonic fluid losses include the gastrointestinal tract, profuse sweating, and renal losses such as with hyperglycemia, mannitol administration, chronic renal failure, and post-obstructive diuresis (urea). Urine sodium and osmolality vary according to the etiology. Extra-renal losses are associated with a urine sodium less than 20 mEq/L and a high urine osmolality. Renal losses are usually associated with a low, normal, or high urine sodium and osmolality.

Hypernatremia with Increased Total Body Sodium

This type of hypernatremia is characterized by an increased total body sodium that exceeds the total body water. When this problem exists, it is most likely iatrogenic in origin. This form of hypernatremia is seen in patients receiving large amounts of sodium bicarbonate during cardiopulmonary resuscitation or lactic acidosis, abortion induced by hypertonic saline, induction of emesis with saline, hemodialysis or peritoneal dialysis, hypertonic infant formula, heat stroke, and sea water drowning. Mild hypernatremia can exist in patients with hyperaldosteronism and Cushing's disease.

Hypernatremia with Normal Total Body Sodium

In this setting, the hypernatremia is associated with water loss without significant sodium loss. This form of hypernatremia is seen in patients with central or nephrogenic diabetes insipidus who fail to respond to thirst stimulation, either due to abnormal thirst response or lack of water. This form is also seen in febrile illnesses in the elderly and in heat stroke where there is an increased insensible loss. In the former, the urine will have an elevated osmolality with a variable urine sodium concentration. If the water loss is renal in origin, both the urine osmolality and sodium concentration may be variable.

Essential hypernatremia is a rare entity, usually associated with a hypothalamic lesion. These patients have an abnormal thirst response to an elevated serum osmolality. An antidiuretic hormone is present although, in some of these patients, vasopressin release is stimulated more by volume depletion as opposed to hyperosmolality.

DIAGNOSIS

Clinical Presentation

A detailed history and physical examination are essential for evaluation of the patient with hypernatremia. A history of systemic disease may be pertinent, especially as related to a recent hospitalization for a central nervous system disorder or renal disease. Information regarding recent exposure to extreme heat or symptoms of infection or stroke are important.

The physical examination should emphasize evaluation of the patient's volume status. Evidence of head trauma, stroke, or severe infarction should be sought. The signs and symptoms of hypernatremia are varied ranging from restlessness alternating with lethargy to seizures. The deleterious effects of hypernatremia are related to the rapidity of development of the abnormality. The cerebrospinal fluid may be xanthrochromic due to secondary capillary rupture.

SIGNS AND SYMPTOMS OF HYPERNATREMIA
In Infants
(Serum Sodium > 150 mEq/L)

High pitched cry	Metabolic acidosis ⎤
Depressed sensorium	Emesis
Hyperactive reflexes	Fever
Muscle twitching	Labored respirations
Seizures	Hemiparesis ⎬ Acute
Hyperglycemia	Spasticity
Hyperkalemia	Babinski
Hypocalcemia	Coma ⎦

In Adults

Depressed sensorium	Seizures
Lethargy	Stupor or Coma
Muscle irritability	Thirst

Laboratory

Electrolytes, BUN, and blood glucose should be drawn. Renal evaluation should include urinary osmolality and electrolytes. Serum osmolality should be calculated and measured.

MANAGEMENT

In general, complete correction of the hyperosmolality should be accomplished over a 48 hour period in order to avoid the development of seizures due to hypotonicity. In the presence of shock, colloid fluid should be given to keep the systolic blood pressure at an adequate level. It must be remembered that most plasma preparations are high in sodium content. After the fluid deficit is estimated, fluid replacement should be instituted. An estimation of the total amount of water deficit can be made by the following formula:

$$H_2O \text{ deficit} = 0.6 \times BW_{kg} \left(1 - \frac{140}{[Na_{obs}]}\right)$$

In all cases, hypotonic fluids are of prime importance. In patients that also have sodium depletion, normal saline preparations should be given to replete intravascular volume and the hypotonic fluids should be administered. Special attention must be given to the possible increase in osmolality by dextrose solutions.

If the patient is severely acidotic, sodium bicarbonate must be given with extreme caution. Serum electrolytes should be measured frequently as well as the serum osmolality. After large volumes of fluid, potassium levels may decrease and should be replaced as needed. Finally, the treatment plan must be modified to accommodate each patient based on the underlying disease.

REFERENCES

Berl T, Anderson RJ, McDonald KM, Schrier RW: Clinical disorders of water metabolism. Kid Int, Vol 10, pp 117–132, 1976

Earley LE, Gottschalk CW: Disorders of water metabolism. *In* Strauss and Welt's Diseases of the Kidney. Vol II, Little, Brown & Co., Boston, Massachusetts, pp 1494, 1499, 1501, 1979

Harrington JT, Cohen JJ: Clinical disorders of urine concentration and dilution. Arch Int Med, Vol 131, pp 810–825, 1973

Levy M: The pathophysiology of sodium balance. Hospital Practice, pp 95–106, 1978

Loeb JN: The hyperosmolar state. New Eng J Med, Vol 290, pp 1184–1187, 1974

Ross, EJ, Christie SBM: Hypernatremia. Medicine, Vol 48, No 6, pp 441–473, 1969

14

UNCOMMON ENDOCRINE-METABOLIC EMERGENCIES

DIABETES INSIPIDUS

Diabetes insipidus is a dramatic disorder of water conservation whereby a debilitating diuresis marked by polydipsia and polyuria results from either:

- An inadequate release of arginine vasopressin in response to physiologic stimuli (neurogenic diabetes insipidus) or
- Renal unresponsiveness to the action of vasopressin (nephrogenic diabetes insipidus).

In either instance the disturbance in water metabolism is the same.

Neurogenic diabetes insipidus can be caused by any lesion that damages the neurohypophysial system and results in failure of antidiuretic hormone production. Permanent diabetes insipidus is associated with destruction of the hypothalamic nuclei or a division of the supraopticoneurohypophysial tract above the median eminence.

Neurogenic diabetes insipidus is associated with primary renal disease (kidney, pyelonephritis, obstructive uropathy, tubular necrosis, cysts), secondary renal lesions (myeloma, sarcoidosis, amyloidosis, sickle cell disease or trait, Sjogren's disease), electrolyte abnormalities (hypokalemia, hypercalcemia), and drugs such as methoxyflurane, lithium, demeclocycline, and amphoterecin B.

The clinical hallmarks are polyuria and polydipsia with little diurnal variation and of such magnitude that normal activity and sleep are almost impossible. Polyuria implies a decrease in the filtered water absorbed by the renal tubule. It can be caused by an alteration in the ability of the tubules to handle water, an osmotic diuresis resulting from impaired solute reabsorption, or both. Thus, the physician must consider, in addition to the causes already mentioned, primary polydipsia, use of diuretics, fluid overload, and diabetes mellitus.

The mild forms of the disorder require no treatment as long as the patient's thirst mechanism is functioning and fluid is available.

Vasopressin-deficient diabetes inspidius can be managed by vasopressin or its synthetic derivatives, agents that stimulate release of antidiuretic hormone, and diuretics that deplete body solutes. Some of these agents are best used concomitantly because their effects are additive.

PHEOCHROMOCYTOMA

Pheochromocytoma occasionally may present as an endocrinologic emergency with the presentation being that of hypertensive crisis. The diagnosis and therapy of this disorder has significantly evolved over the past decade. Since the clinical expressions are so variable the diagnosis of this disorder must begin with high suspicion.

Pheochromocytoma may occur at any age and most patients have a characteristic history suggesting episodic attacks which clinically express themselves with headache, sweating, anxiety, hypertension, or palpitations.

The most dramatic presentation of this disorder usually relates to the hypertensive crisis and the possible complications of this including myocardial infarction, cerebrovascular accident, dissecting aneurysm, or congestive heart failure.

Treatment of hypertensive crises caused by pheochromocytoma revolves around the use of adrenergic-blocking drugs of the alpha-antagonist category. Phentolamine (Regitine®) is a short-acting drug which may be administered either orally or intervenously. Its use for pre-operative or chronic therapy is rarely, if ever, indicated, and its major usefulness is for acute control of hypertensive crises.

The reader is referred to the references for a more detailed discussion of diabetes insipidus, pheochromocytoma, and hypertensive crisis.

REFERENCES

Manger WM, Gifford RW: Pheochromocytoma: Diagnosis and management. New York State Journal of Medicine, p 216, February 1980

Rush DR, Hamburger SL: Management of diabetes insipidus. Family Practice Recertification, Vol 3, p 10, 1981

Weitzman R, Kleeman CR: Water metabolism and the neurohypophysial hormones. *In* Bondy PK, Rosenberg LE (eds): Metabolic Control and Disease, 8th ed. W.B. Saunders Co., Philadelphia, Pennsylvania, p 1241, 1980

DIAGNOSTIC SYLLABUS FOR ENDOCRINE AND METABOLIC EMERGENCIES

DIAGNOSTIC SYLLABUS

Metabolic problems are frequently encountered within the province of the emergency department. The manifestations of such disorders are legion. In cases of acute renal or pulmonary failure, ingestion of toxins, and diabetic coma, the nature of the metabolic derangement can frequently be diagnosed from the history, physical examination, and laboratory data base. However, when a metabolic disturbance is expressed as a focal neurological lesion, coma, seizure disorder, cardiac arrest, myopathy, or non-specific symptom complex, the diagnosis may be much more difficult. In such cases, if a systematic approach to metabolic problems is not employed, the disease may go undiagnosed and, hence, untreated.

To ensure rapid institution of appropriate therapy for derangements of metabolic homeostasis, the emergency physician must be familiar with a myriad of disorders and be able to distinguish among them using a paucity of quickly available laboratory data.

I. METABOLIC EMERGENCIES: IMPORTANCE OF EARLY DIAGNOSIS

A. Metabolic derangements can serve as diagnostic clues to the presence of:

1. Toxic ingestions
2. Hemodynamic compromise
3. Respiratory failure

4. Postictal states
5. Other (SIADH, Addisonian crisis, hypothyroidism, etc.)

B. Therapeutic decisions depend upon rapid diagnosis:

1. Choice of IV fluids
2. Oral therapy
3. Dextrose therapy
4. ETOH therapy (i.e., in ethylene glycol ingestion)
5. Insulin therapy
6. Others (dialysis, hemoperfusion with charcoal, etc.)

C. Disposition and triage of patients depend upon early recognition of nature and severity of metabolic disturbance:

1. ICU, CCU vs. dialysis
2. Invasive vs. non-invasive monitoring

II. CLINICAL CONDITIONS: METABOLIC PROBLEMS

A. Metabolic disorders in the emergency department:

1. Shock (lactic acidosis, rhabdomyolysis, hyperkalemia, hyperphosphatemia, alcohol or drug ingestion, respiratory alkalosis, or acidosis)
2. Cardiopulmonary arrest (hypo- or hyperkalemia, lactic acidosis, hypocalcemia in EM dissociation, etc.)
3. Seizures (hyponatremia, hypocalcemia, hypomagnesemia, hypoglycemia, hyperosmolar states, rhabdomyolysis, etc.)
4. Coma (diabetic or alcoholic ketoacidosis, hyperosmolar nonketotic coma, hyponatremia, hypoglycemia, hyperammonemia, etc.)
5. Respiratory failure (hypercapnia, CO_2 narcosis, etc.)
6. Toxic ingestion (methanol, ethylene glycol, paraldehyde, ethanol, etc.)

III. EMERGENCY ROOM BATTERY (ERB)

Emergency room battery (ERB) is a conceptual, quasi-algorithmic scheme that is intended to guide the emergency room physician in the diagnosis and evaluation of acute metabolic emergencies.

The ERB framework (ERB-6, ERB-9, ERB-15, ERB-18, ERB-20—number represents how many lab tests are included in battery) is organized in hierarchical fashion to facilitate the diagnosis of increasingly complex and/or unusual metabolic derangements. The laboratory tests included in the ERBs include only those available on a STAT basis.

A. ERB-6—Na, K, Cl, CO_2, Glucose, BUN

This is the minimal and initial diagnostic data base for the evaluation of metabolic disorders in coma, seizures, acute renal failure, nonketotic hyperosmolar coma, pre-renal azotemia, high anion gap (i.e., organic acid) acidoses, adrenocortical insufficiency, toxic ingestions, and in non-specific presentations.

NOTE: The ERB-6 is almost always used in conjunction with other lab tests (especially ABGs) in order to fully elucidate the exact nature of a metabolic disturbance.

B. ERB-9 = ERB-6 + pH, pCO_2, pO_2

The ERB-9 is needed for nearly all of the entities listed under ERB-6 plus all cases of suspected mixed acid-base disorders, respiratory distress, as well as for non-metabolic disorders such as asthma, pulmonary embolism, and pulmonary edema.

C. ERB-15 = ERB-9 + U_{Na}, U_{Cl}, $U_{ketones}$, $U_{glucose}$, U_{osm}, P_{osm}

The ERB-15 is needed for many of the conditions listed under ERB-6 and ERB-9, as well as for the **complete** and **rapid** evaluation (or confirmation) of diabetic ketoacidosis, alcoholic ketoacidosis (false negative nitroprusside reaction for ketones is common), SIADH (syndrome of inappropriate ADH can easily be diagnosed as U_{osm} is inappropriately concentrated with respect to P_{osm}), for distinguishing ATN from pre-renal azotemia, for differentiating "saline-responsive" vs. "saline-resistant" (U_{Cl}) metabolic alkalosis, and for a clue (P_{osm}) to the presence of ETOH, methanol, or ethylene glycol ingestions.

D. ERB-18 = ERB-15 + Ca, PO_4, Mg

For many of the conditions listed under other ERBs (i.e., DKA, ETOH withdrawal, renal failure, etc.) and especially when myoirritability (i.e., positive Chvostek's or Trousseau's Syndrome), EM (electromechanical) dissociation, rhabdomyolysis (i.e., elevated PO_4 and decreased Ca), lactic acidosis (elevated PO_4), starvation, metastatic CA (elevated Ca), cardiomyopathy, or hypophosphatemia is present or suspected.

E. ERB-20 = ERB-18 + U_{Cr}, P_{Cr}

For renal disorders, assessment of volume status, and in other conditions when RFI (Renal Failure Index) may be helpful (RFI discussed below).

IV. DIAGNOSTIC TOOLS FOR RAPID EVALUATION OF METABOLIC DISORDERS

A. Arterial Blood Gas interpretation

NINE CATEGORIES OF ACID-BASE DISTURBANCE AS DEFINED BY THE PCO₂ AND BICARBONATE LEVELS

PCO₂	Bicarbonate (mEq/liter)		
	< 21	*21–26*	*> 26*
> 45	Combined metabolic and respiratory acidosis	Respiratory acidosis	Metabolic alkalosis and respiratory acidosis
35–45	Metabolic acidosis	Normal	Metabolic alkalosis
< 35	Metabolic acidosis and respiratory alkalosis	Respiratory alkalosis	Combined metabolic and respiratory alkalosis

B. BUN/Cr Ratio

When ratio >15:1, this suggests **pre-renal azotemia** (i.e., dehydration or pre-renal hypoperfusion on some other basis).

C. Use of the renal failure index (RFI) and fractional excretion of sodium RE_{Na}

$$RFI = \frac{U_{Na}}{U_{Cr}/P_{Cr}} \; ; \; FE_{Na} = \frac{U_{Na}/P_{Na}}{U_{Cr}/P_{Cr}}$$

If RFI < 1: Pre-renal causes
If RFI > 1: ATN, vascular, or postrenal causes

D. Interpretation of Urinary Electrolytes

U_{Na}.   In general, a healthy (i.e., non-ATN) kidney is able to conserve sodium. Therefore, in the oliguric patient (anuria is seen almost *only* in postrenal **obstruction**) who has an elevated BUN and Cr, a **pre-renal** picture will be characterized by a low U_{Na} (i.e., < 20meg/L), whereas the ATN picture will be characterized by high U_{Na} (i.e., > 40). NOTE: Diuretics can make a pre-renal picture look like ATN because they increase U_{Na} excretion (in such cases use RFI or FE_{Na} to refine diagnosis).

U_{Cr}.   In general, a healthy kidney is able to concentrate creatinine (Cr) in the urine, whereas a diseased (i.e., ATN, etc.) kidney will excrete Cr at about the same concentration as it is in the plasma.

Therefore, a **pre-renal** picture is characterized by:

$$U_{Cr}/P_{Cr} > 20:1$$

whereas an ATN picture is characterized by:

$$U_{Cr}/P_{Cr} = 1:1$$

U_{Cl}. Value lies in distinguishing among etiologies in metabolic alkalosis. **Volume contraction** (i.e., NG suction, diuretic therapy, dehydration) alkalosis will be characterized by avid NaCl reabsorption, and, therefore, the U_{Cl} will be low (i.e., > 10meg/L).

Metabolic alkalosis caused by **hyperadrenal** states (i.e., increased serum cortisol and/or mineralocorticoids which cause increased Na for K and H+ exchange distally) is usually characterized by U_{Cl} > 10meg.

U_{osm}. In general, a diseased kidney will not be able to concentrate well, and so in the oliguric patient with elevated BUN and Cr, an isosmotic urine suggests ATN, and a concentrated urine (i.e., > 550osm) suggests **pre-renal** causes. Also, the U_{osm} is probably the most important test for ascertaining the diagnosis of SIADH. If the $U_{osm} > P_{osm}$ in the patient who is severely hyponatremic and hypoosmolar, this virtually confirms the diagnosis of SIADH. Actually, any U_{osm} that is not **maximally dilute** (i.e., 50–85 mosm/L) in a patient with hyponatremia and hypo-osmolarity is suggestive of SIADH.

E. Serum Osmolality

Serum osmolality can be both **calculated** and **measured.**
If calculated:

$$S_{osm} = 2 \times Na + Glucose/18 + BUN/3$$

If measured:

$$S_{osm} \text{ CALCULATED } S_{osm}$$

then molecules (i.e., other than Na, BUN, and glucose) with significant osmotic properties are present in the serum. In general, these

---

VALUE OF THE DETERMINATION OF URINARY CHLORIDE CONCENTRATION IN THE DIFFERENTIAL DIAGNOSIS OF METABOLIC ALKALOSIS

Saline-Responsive U_{Cl} less than 10meg/L	*Saline-Resistant* U_{Cl} greater than 10meg/L
• Loss of gastric secretions (i.e., vomiting or nasogastric suction) • Diuretic therapy	• Primary aldosteronism • Cushing's disease • Adrenocorticotrophic hormone (ACTH) producing tumors • Severe potassium depletion • Steroid therapy

might be ETOH (a 25 mosm difference between calculated and measured serum osmolality would be compatible with an ETOH level of 100–120 mg percent), methanol, ethylene glycol, or mannitol. Therefore, patients whose osm cannot be explained by ETOH level should be suspected of having ingested one of the above-mentioned toxins.

F. Winter's Formula

Winter's formula is a quick way to measure appropriateness of respiratory response (i.e., hyper- or hypoventilation) to a metabolic disturbance.

As a rule:

If $pCO_2 = 1.5$ (total serum CO_2) + 8.3, appropriate respiratory compensation is present.

If $pCO_2 < 1.5$ (total serum CO_2) + 8.3, then a primary respiratory alkalosis is superimposed on metabolic disturbance.

If $pCO_2 > 1.5$ (total serum CO_2) + 8.3, then a primary respiratory acidosis is superimposed on metabolic disturbance.

G. Bypassing Henderson-Hasselbalch Equation

A simple method reported in JACEP (Kamens et. al.) that allows you to *estimate* serum bicarb (HCO_3) concentration from the ABG values pH, pCO_2 is shown on page 125.

V. ANION GAP

$$Na^+ - (Cl^- + HCO_3^-) = AG$$

A. Introduction

NOTE: This is one of the most important diagnostic tools to measure for the evaluation of acute metabolic emergencies.

The anion gap is a calculation of diagnostic convenience. There is, of course, no true anion gap since positive and negative charges in the blood must be equal. However, the principal cation of the blood, sodium (Na), exceeds the sum of the principal anions, chloride and bicarbonate, by about 12 ± 2 meg/L in normal persons. The additional, or so-called unmeasured, anions include albumin (which is an anion at physiologic pH) and other metabolites such as sulfate, phosphates, and small amounts of organic acids. When metabolic acids are generated and added to the body fluid, the hydrogen ion of the acid destroys bicarbonate, and if the anion associated with the proton (i.e., hydrogen) is any other than chlo-

ESTIMATING BICARBONATE ION CONCENTRATION

Range	$[HCO_3-]/pCO_2$ Estimate	Examples $[HCO_3-]/pCO_2$ from pH	Estimated $[HCO_3-]$
Severe acidemia (7.00 > pH)	0.20	if pH = 6.89 $$\frac{[HCO_3-]}{pCO_2} = 0.20$$	$[HCO_3-]$ = 20% of pCO_2
Mild—Moderate Acidemia (7.00 ≤ pH ≤ 7.40)	(pH − 7) + 0.20	if pH = 7.[25] $$0.25 + 0.20 = 0.45$$ $$\frac{[HCO_3-]}{pCO_2} = 0.45$$	$[HCO_3-]$ = 45% of pCO_2
Alkalemia (pH > 7.40)	2[(pH − 7) − 0.10]	if pH = 7.[60] $$0.60 - 0.10 = 0.50$$ $$2 \times 0.50 = 1.00$$ $$\frac{[HCO_3-]}{pCO_2} = 1.00$$	$[HCO_3-]$ = 100% of pCO_2

Kamens DR, et al: Circumventing the Henderson-Hasselbalch equation. JACEP, Vol 8, No 11, p 462, November 1979 ride, the sum of chloride and bicarbonate must fall, thereby increasing the anion gap.

B. Differential Diagnosis of Elevated and Reduced Anion Gap

The most important thing about the anion gap is for the emergency physician to get in the habit of using this simple and revealing calculation on a routine basis. Failure to employ this diagnostic tool may allow any of the following to go undetected:

1. Organic acidosis
2. Toxin-induced acidoses
3. Severe alkalemia
4. Mixed acid-base disturbances.

A reduced anion gap may also be an important finding and is frequently the first clue in the ER that cirrhosis, lithium toxicity, hypercalcemia, hypermagnesemia, or multiple myeloma is present.

C. Anion Gap and Alkalemia

NOTE: This is a relatively new, but relevant, discovery.

$$\text{Anion gap} = Na^+ - (Cl^- + HCO_3^-) = AG$$

When investigating the cause of an elevated anion gap (AG), the ER clinician routinely seeks evidence for the presence of lactic acidosis, ASA ingestion, advanced renal failure, methanol, paraldehyde, or ethylene glycol ingestion, diabetic ketoacidosis (DKA), or alcoholic ketoacidosis.

Frequently, however, consideration is not given to the possibility that changes in unmeasured anions, originating from plasma proteins, may have contributed to the increase in anion gap. It is now well established that increases in unmeasured anions may result from alkalemia-induced elevations in the net negative charge of plasma proteins.

D. Anion Gap, Serum Proteins, and Alkalemia

$$AG = Na - (Cl + HCO_3)$$

AG = largely reflects organic sulfates, phosphates, and negatively charged serum proteins, of which albumin is the most important.

$$\text{Albumin-H} \xrightarrow{\quad\text{Alkalemia}\quad} \text{Albumin}^- + H^+$$

$$\text{Albumin}^- \uparrow \longrightarrow \uparrow \quad \text{ANION GAP}$$

E. Anion Gap: Some Pearls

Recognize that a **normal measured serum** HCO_3 does *not* mean that there is not a **metabolic acidosis** present. If there is a **pre-existing metabolic alkalosis** (i.e., vomiting, diuretics, ETOH'ism, metabolic compensation for respiratory acidosis, etc.), the serum HCO_3 will be elevated *at first*, and then can *fall to a normal range* (or perhaps lower) in the presence of a super-imposed metabolic acidosis.

The presence of a pre-existing metabolic alkalosis can be detected using the AG.

$$\Delta\ AG\ =\ AG(calculated)\ -\ AG(normal, i.e., 12)$$

$$\Delta\ HCO_3\ =\ HCO_3\ (expected—i.e.,\ 24\ meg)\ -\ HCO_3(measured)$$

If:

$$\Delta\ AG\ >\ \Delta\ HCO_3$$

suspect a metabolic acidosis that has been superimposed on a pre-existing metabolic *alkalosis*.

F. Anion Gap: Extended Data Base (i.e., further lab work-up in ER)

EXTENDED DATA BASE FOR EVALUATION OF ELEVATED ANION GAP

1. **DKA:** Urine ketones, serum ketones, serum K^+, serum PO_4, glucose, lactate level, ABG.
2. **Alcoholic ketosis**
   - Urine ketones (but note that the nitroprusside reagent, Acetest, may be entirely negative because this kind of acidosis is characteristically a B-OH butyric acidosis; serum ketones are usually positive)
   - Glucose (especially important, since this syndrome may be accompanied by hypoglycemia, i.e., hypoglycemic ketoacidotic coma)
   - Urine glucose (almost always negative in this kind of ketoacidosis).
3. **Lactic acidosis**
   - Lactate level, K^+; may need to draw CN^-, methemoglobin, or carboxyhemoglobin level for "unexplained" cases of lactic acidosis
   - In cases of quickly resolving LA, consider generalized motor seizures as likely etiology and initiate work-up as needed.
4. **Salicyclate overdose:** Salicyclate level, ABGs and lactate level (if acidosis is very severe; salicyclates may uncouple oxidative phosphorylation and lead to LA).

5. **Ethylene glycol ingestion:** Blood level, serum osmolality, urinalysis, and renal work-up.
6. **Methanol:** Blood level, serum osmolality.
7. **Paraldehyde**
8. **Alkalemia:** Work up various etiologies.

G. Low Anion Gap: Differential Diagnosis

Causes of Low Anion Gap
1. Reduced concentration of unmeasured anions
   - Dilution
   - Hypoalbuminemia
2. Systematic underestimation of serum sodium
   - Hypernatremia (severe)
   - Hyperviscosity
3. Systematic overestimation of serum chloride
   - Bromism
4. Retained non-sodium cations
   - Paraproteinemia
   - Hypercalcemia, hypermagnesemia, lithium toxicity

H. Anion Gap and Metabolic Acidosis

1. Lactic Acidosis (Most Common Cause of Elevated AG)

Causes of Lactic Acidosis
1. Inadequate Oxygen Delivery
   - Cardiac arrest
   - Shock states
   - Profound anemia
   - Hypoxemia

2. Failure to utilize oxygen
   - Phenformin
   - Ethanol
   - Diabetic ketoacidosis
   - Leukemia and lymphoma
   - INH overdose

3. Others
   - Hepatic cirrhosis
   - Pregnancy
   - Pancreatitis
   - Seizures
   - CRF

DIFFERENTIAL DIAGNOSIS OF METABOLIC ACIDOSIS

Normal Anion Gap (Hyperchloremic)	*Increased Anion Gap*
Gastrointestinal loss of HCO₃	**Increased Acid Production**

Normal Anion Gap (Hyperchloremic)

Gastrointestinal loss of HCO₃
- Diarrhea
- Ureterosigmoidostomy
- Anion-exchange resin
- Small bowel drainage

Renal loss of HCO₃
- Carbonic anhydrase inhibitors
- Renal Tubular Acidosis (RTA)

Miscellaneous
- Dilutional acidosis
- Hyperalimentation acidosis

Increased Anion Gap

Increased Acid Production
- Diabetic ketoacidosis
- Lactic acidosis
- Starvation
- Alcoholic ketoacidosis
- Inborn errors of metabolism

Ingestion of toxins
- Salicylate overdose
- Paraldehyde poisoning
- Methanol ingestion
- Ethylene glycol ingestion

Acute or Chronic Renal Failure

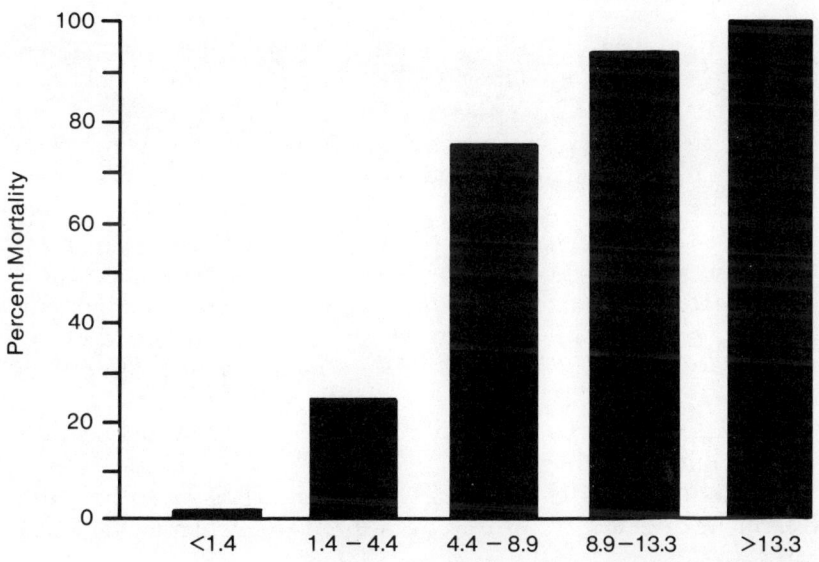

The relationship with mortality—the prognostic significance of initial arterial lactate concentration in 52 patients with shock of various etiologies is shown. The mortality in patients with a lactate level of 1.4 to 4.4 mMoles/liter (22%) was significantly less than when the lactate levels were between 4.4 and 8.9 mMoles/liter (78%). (Perets DI: Ann NY Acad Sci, Vol 119, p 1133, 1965)

2. Prognostic Features of Lactic Acidosis

VI. CASE PRESENTATIONS

A. Estimating Bicarbonate Ion

A 26 year-old white male with history of JODM presents to the ER with SOB, nausea, vomiting, and abdominal pain. PE reveals a conscious patient who is slightly confused with a BP of 110/70, R = 28, T = 36.5, and HR = 110. One liter of .9NS is started. ABGs return in four minutes (calculated bicarb not ordered) with pH = 7.08, $pCO_2 = 13$, and $pO_2 = 142$.

(Formula for estimating bicarb concentration—see IV. G.)
For pH between 7.00 and 7.40:

$$(pH - 7.00) + .20 \times pCO_2 = HCO_3$$
$$(7.08 - 7.00) + .20 = .28$$
$$.28 \times 13 = 3.64 = \text{estimated } HCO_3$$

ERB-6 returns with measured $HCO_3 = 4$.

B. Lactic Acidosis Presenting as Respiratory Problem

A 60 year-old white male presents to the Emanuel Hospital Emergency Department with a depressed LOC. He appears to be in moderate respiratory distress. Vital signs reveal that BP = 105/70, RR = 22, Temp = 37.5, and HR = 120. Cardiac exam reveals an S_3 and pulmonary exam reveals diffuse rhonchi and rales bilaterally, posteriorly. A history of COPD is obtained. Initial lab data includes ABG: pH = 7.25, pCO_2 - 57, pO_2 = 52. (A medical resident is called to see the patient and makes a "diagnosis" of acute respiratory failure with respiratory acidosis.) Additional lab values return in the ER: Na = 136, Cl = 90, HCO_3 = 25, K = 4.0, BUN = 40, Cr = 1.6. (Anion gap elevated = 21.) Elevated AG suggests metabolic acidosis is the primary metabolic derangement. Lactic acid is drawn and elevated (10.6 mmole/L). The patient is treated with diuretics and morphine for cardiac failure (low output state) and pulmonary edema (CXR confirms). Repeat gases shortly after treatment show pH = 7.35, pCO_2 = 54, pO_2 = 60. HCO_3 = 30. This represents patient's baseline state (i.e., chronic respiratory acidosis with metabolic compensation).

In summary, this is a case in which the acidosis resolved with treatment directed at low output failure rather than at the respiratory system.

ALSO NOTE:

$$\Delta AG = 21 - 12 = 9$$
$$\Delta HCO_3 = 24 - 25 = (-1)$$
$\Delta AG > \Delta HCO_3$ giving a clue to the presence of pre-existing metabolic alkalosis

C. Severe Acidosis and Hyperkalemia

An 80 year-old white male, who is taking digoxin and diuretics, is brought to the Good Samaritan ER with severe SOB, tachypnea, and mental confusion. Vital signs: Temp = 38.2 C, HR = 110, RR = 28, BP = 180/105. Physical exam reveals a dehydrated, dyspneic patient, with rhonchi and rales at the right lower lung base. CXR reveals an infiltrate and an EKG strip shows occasional focal PVCs. The patient is started on 3L O_2 and the following ERB results return: pH = 7.16, pO_2 = 60, pCO_2 = 54, Na = 135, C1 = 108, CO_2 = 21, K = 7.1, BUN = 90, Cr = 2.2, U_{Na} = 48, U_{Cr} = 118, U_{osm} = 440, Anion gap = 8.

$$\text{RFI (Renal Failure Index)} = \frac{U_{Na}}{U_{Cr}/P_{Cr}} = \frac{48}{118/2.2} = .94$$

Because the RFI was less than 1 (and also because the BUN/Cr was greater than 20), the patient was presumed to have pre-renal azotemia; 2 amps (110 mEq) of $NaHCO_3$, 25u regular insulin, and 1000 ccs $D_{10}W$ (i.e., 100 gms glucose) were administered in the ER. The patient improved clinically and repeat ERB revealed: K = 5.9; pH = 7.28, pO_2 = 60, pCO_2 = 50.

NOTE: This patient has a primary hyperchloremic (non AG) metabolic acidosis superimposed on a chronic respiratory acidosis (presumably 2° COPD). In distinguishing among the causes of the acidoses it is important to note:

1. That a pCO_2 = 54 will not explain a pH = 7.16
2. That while a HCO_3 = 21 does not "immediately suggest a significant metabolic acidosis, it is compatible with this diagnosis if you assume that a patient has a chronically elevated HCO_3 (35–40 mEq) as a compensatory response to a chronic respiratory acidosis.

CONCLUSION: Do not assume normal measured serum HCO rules out.

The RFI (calculated from values obtained in the ER) was useful in ascertaining that this patient's elevated BUN, Cr, and potassium, as well as the oliguria and metabolic acidosis, were on the basis of a pre-renal azotemia rather than ATN. Once this had been determined, a sodium load ($NaHCO_3$) could be administered without much fear of fluid overload. CONCLUSION: Obtaining urinary diagnostic indices in the ER can be quite helpful in deciding initial fluid therapy and can frequently anticipate or rule out the necessity for dialysis.

D. Respiratory Acidosis in Pulmonary Edema

A 60 year-old white male with a previous history of CHF presents to the University of Chicago Hospitals and Clinics ER with a CC:

SOB. Vital signs: BP = 180/100, R = 24, T = 37°, and HR = 115. Physical exam reveals bibasilar rales and an S_3 gallop. ABGs are drawn at time of admission and patient is subsequently given 6 mg morphine sulfate IV. Initial (i.e., pre-therapy) ABGs return: pH = 7.27, pCO_2 = 52, pO_2 = 64 (anion gap from ERB-6 is WNL). Patient improves dramatically and repeat gases show pH = 7.36, pCO_2 = 38, pO_2 = 79.

COMMENT: When hypercapnia and acute respiratory acidosis are caused by alveolar edema and bronchoconstriction 2° to LV failure, administration of MS—despite the fact that it is a respiratory depressant—is usually safe and effective.

E. Metabolic Derangement Presenting as Cardiac Arrest

A 58 year-old white male with a previous history of CAD collapses suddenly at home, without a prodrome of chest pain, nausea, or diaphoresis. He is taking digoxin and diuretics but no K supplementation. The patient is successfully resuscitated by the paramedics, who have intubated him and given him 1 amp of $NaHCO_3$ about 30 minutes before arrival at the Providence Hospital ER. The patient was cardioverted from ventricular fibrillation to NSR and started on a lidocaine drip by the paramedics. Upon admission to the ER he is perfusing well: BP = 120/70, Resp rate (artificial ventilation), and HR = 86. EKG reveals old AMI with multifocal PVCs. First lab data to return are ABGs: pH = 7.62, pCO_2 = 30, and pO_2 = 160 (50% FiO_2). Calculated serum bicarb is 31 mEq/L. On the basis of combined primary metabolic and respiratory alkalosis, patient is presumed to be hypokalemic and volume contracted, probably secondary to diuretic therapy. Therefore, 10 mEq KCl is added to IV to run over observation period (45 minutes) in ER. ERB-6 returns 30 minutes after arrival and shows: Na = 139, Cl = 90, CO_2 = 31, K = 2.9, BUN = 37, Cr = 1.1, AG = 18 (lactate not measured). Patient's frequent PVCs respond to KCl therapy.

COMMENT: If the ER physician is quick on his/her feet, he/she can recognize that metabolic alkalosis in the arrest patient might be the first tip-off of a volume contraction, hypokalemic metabolic alkalosis. If the ventricular arrhythmia appears refractory to suppressive therapy, quick administration of KCl may be warranted. This patient's elevated AG probably reflects alkalemia rather than acidosis. The elevated BUN/Cr ratio argues convincingly for prerenal azotemia which, in this case, was probably induced by diuretic therapy.

F. Necessity of Measuring Anion Gap in Mixed Acid-Base Disorders

A 35-year-old white female presents to the University of Oregon Health Sciences Center ER after four days of heavy alcohol ingestion and persistent vomiting. On admission she is confused, lethargic, and responds to questions inappropriately. There is no odor of alcohol or ammonia. ABGs reveal pH $= 7.52$, $pCO_2 = 28$, and $pO_2 = 90$. Based upon this data, the medical intern in the ER makes a "diagnosis" of acute respiratory alkalosis. The ERB-6 returns and reveals a BUN $= 28$, Cr $= 2.3$, Na $= 129$, Cl $= 78$, K $= 3.0$, and $HCO_3 = 25$. With this additional information, the intern "confirms" a diagnosis of acute respiratory alkalosis with incomplete metabolic compensation. The ER resident is called to see the patient. He calculates the AG (26), which suggests an organic acidosis. Serum lactate is measured (elevated 13.9 mmoles/L), urinary ketones $= 1+$, and serum ketones positive 1:8.

COMMENT: What initially appeared to be a simple respiratory alkalosis is actually a complicated, mixed acid-base disturbance requiring urgent therapy. This patient had both a primary respiratory and metabolic alkalosis (2° to vomiting) and superimposed upon these were alcoholic ketoacidosis and alcohol-induced acidosis. This patient resolved all her metabolic derangements with the vigorous administration of D_5NS and KCl.

NOTE: The initial measured serum bicarbonate (HCO_3) was 25 mEq/L (i.e., within the normal range), despite a significant lactic and ketoacidosis. How is this explained? Presumably, there was a significant primary metabolic alkalosis (2° to vomiting, as explained above) which raised the bicarb to 35 mEq/L, a value which was then titrated down into the normal range by the presence of these two organic acids.

G. Hypothermia, Hypoglycemia, Hypotension

A 43 year-old white female with a history of metastatic breast Ca presents to the Emanuel Hospital ER with an altered mental status and CC: weakness, nausea, and abdominal pain. PE reveals BP $= 88/50$, R $= 26$, HR $= 110$, and T $= 35.4°$. The rest of the exam is non-contributory. Patient is observed in the ER and ERB-6 returns: Glucose $= 38$ mg/100 ml, BUN $= 34$, Na $= 132$, $CO_2 = 22$, Cl $= 100$, and K $= 4.9$. The patient is given 50 cc of 50% $D_{50}W$ as well as volume replacement with .9NS with significant improvement in level of consciousness and slight increase in body temperature. A complete ERB-18 is collected: ABGs show pH $= 7.48$, $pCO_2 = 82$. Ca, PO_4 and mg are WNL. $U_{Cl} = 20$ mEq, $U_{Na} = 40$, U_{ket} and U_{glu} are negative. $U_{Cr} = 30$, $P_{Cr} = 1.1$ (RFI greater than 1). Patient is admitted to medical wards where, within the next 18 hours, she has two more episodes of profound, sudden hypoglycemia, as well as persistent hypotension. She has two cardiac arrests and finally dies despite vigorous therapy.

COMMENT: At autopsy, this patient had an empty sella syndrome, with no remnants of pituitary tissue. Despite persistent hypotension (2° to NaCl loss because of hypocortisolism), repeat bouts of hypoglycemia (also a result of inadequate glucocorticoids), and excessive urinary Na and Cl losses, the diagnosis of Addisonian crisis was not made. This patient expired because steroids were never included in her therapeutic management.

H. Metabolic Disturbance Presenting as Focal Neurological Lesion

A 60 year-old black female with CRF and AODM, and who is taking oral hypoglycemia medication, is brought to the Emanual ER with a markedly depressed mental status and left-sided hemiparesis. PE reveals vital signs: T = 35.8, R = 24, P = 110, BP = 212/118. Neuro exam demonstrates a profound left-sided hemiparesis, expressive aphasia, and the presence of a Babinski reflex on the left. Initial diagnostic impression in the ER is intracerebral hemorrhage (hypertensive). ERB-6 returns: Glucose = 26 mg/100 ml and otherwise normal electrolytes. Patient's entire neurological deficit resolves after administration of 50 cc of 50% glucose IV.

COMMENT: Focal neurological lesions (deficits and seizures) can result from metabolic derangements.

I. Metabolic Disturbance Presenting as Focal Neurological Lesion

An 83 year-old black male with a history of oral hypoglycemic use and AODM is admitted to the University of Chicago ER with a depressed LOC and dense right-sided hemiparesis. VS reveal BP = 160/80, HR = 120, T = 38.2, and R = 26. The initial diagnostic impression is left middle cerebral artery thromboembolic infarction. ERB-6 returns: Glucose = 1190 mg/100 ml; remainder of studies are consistent with diagnosis of non-ketotic hyperosmolar coma. Patient is treated with insulin, hydration, and appropriate electrolyte replacement. Neurological status returns to baseline, including complete resolution of hemiparesis.

J. Mixed Metabolic Derangements

A 66 year-old white male alcoholic is brought to the University of Chicago ER comatose and diaphoretic. Vital signs are T = 36.2, R = 22, H.R. = 120, BP = 120/70. Cardiac and lung exam are noncontributory, but abdominal exam reveals hepatomegaly. Patient is given 200 mg thiamine IV and 50 cc $D_{50}W$, and quickly regains consciousness. ERB-6 (drawn before therapy) reveals glucose = 39, BUN = 6, Na = 139, K = 5.2, Cl = 100, CO_2 = 20. Initial diagnostic impression is hypoglycemia 2° depleted hepatic glycogen stores. Despite glucose therapy, patient's mental status remains somewhat

LABORATORY SUMMARY OF NONDIABETIC ALCOHOLIC PATIENTS WITH HYPOGLYCEMIC KETOACIDOTIC COMA

Case	Arterial pH	Serum Acetest for Ketones	Urine Acetest for Ketones	Serum Glucose (mg/dl) Initial	Discharge	Serum Bicarbonate (mEq/liter) (normal 24–30) Initial	Discharge	Lactic Acid, Arterial (mEq per liter) (normal .5–1.5)	Serum β-hydroxybutyrate (mEq per liter) (normal<.05)	Anion Gap (Na+K−) [Cl+HCO₂]	Serum Bilirubin (mg/dl)	Serum Insulin (µU/ml)	SGOT (IU/liter) (normal<17)
1	7.16	+	+	25	105	14	21	2.6	9.8	27	1.0	..	55
2	7.18	+	+	21	120	15	20	2.3	..	21	0.8	3	40
3	7.23	−	−	27	125	17	24	..	7.3	22	0.7	..	35
4	7.19	−	−	21	110	13	22	2.2	8.5	29	1.1	5	30
5	7.18	+	+	19	105	15	23	2.4	5.9	24	0.9	2	31
Mean	7.19	..	..	23	..	15	..	2.4	7.9	25	0.9	3	38

Platia EZ, Hsu TH: Hypoglycemic coma with ketoacidosis in nondiabetic adults. West J Med, Vol 131, No 4, p 272, October 1981 unclear. Reassessment of problem shows an AG of 19, suggesting organic acidosis. ABGs show pH = 7.28, pCO_2 = 35, pO_2 = 85; Urine ketones = 2 + and serum ketones are positive at 1:4. Lactate, salicylates, and serum osm are WNL. Patient has hypoglycemia alcoholic ketoacidotic coma.

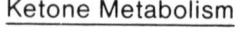

Ketone Metabolism

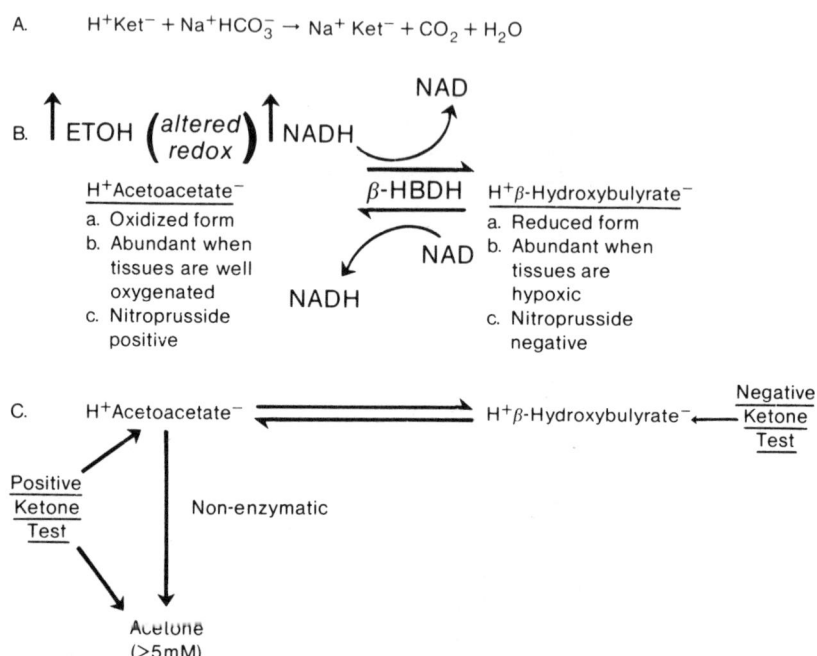

Ketone Metabolism.

K. Acute Hyponatremia

A 48 year-old white male with a previous psychiatric history and mild hypertension (recently started on a thiazide diuretic) is brought to the Portland V.A. ER in a postictal state after having had two generalized seizures. The paramedic described the seizures as beginning at the left arm, moving to the left leg, and then generalizing. Dilantin loading is started in the ER (at 25 mg/min) but despite this patient has another seizure. ERB-18 returns with following results: Na = 116, K = 2.8, CO_2 = 30, Cl = 80, BUN = 28; ABGs show pH = 7.52, pCO_2 = 32, pO_2 = 100; Ca, PO_4, and Mg are WNL. U_{Na} = 6, U_{osm} = 420, Serum $_{osm}$ = 245. On the basis of hyponatremia and inappropriate urinary concentration in the face of serum hypo-osmolality, a diagnosis of SIADH is made. Because of continued seizures 3% saline and diuresis with 20 mg of furosemide is initiated.

DIFFERENTIAL DIAGNOSIS OF HYPONATREMIA WITH NORMAL HYDRATION

	Inappropriate-ADH Secretion	Hypopituitarism	Hypothyroidism	Diuretic-Induced	Chlorpropamide-Induced	Polydipsic Vomiting
Creatinine clearance	Normal or ↑	Normal or slightly ↓	Normal or slightly ↓	Normal or slightly ↓	Normal or ↑	Normal or ↓
Serum K	Normal	Normal	Normal		Normal	↓
Serum HCO₃⁻	Normal	Normal	Normal	↑ Early, ↓ Later	Normal	↑
Urine Na⁺	↑	↑	↓	↑ Early, ↓ Later	↑	↓
Urine osmolality	↑	↑	↑		↑	↑
Metapyrone response	Normal	↓	Normal	Normal	Normal	Normal
H₂O load response	↓	↓	Delayed	Normal	Delayed	Normal
Correction	H₂O restriction	Cortisol	Thyroid	Withdraw diuretics or ↑ K⁺ intake	Withdraw chlorpropamide	NaCl, KCl, and H₂O restriction

Adapted from Berl T, et al: Clinical disorders of water metabolism. Kidney Int, Vol 10, No 117, 1976

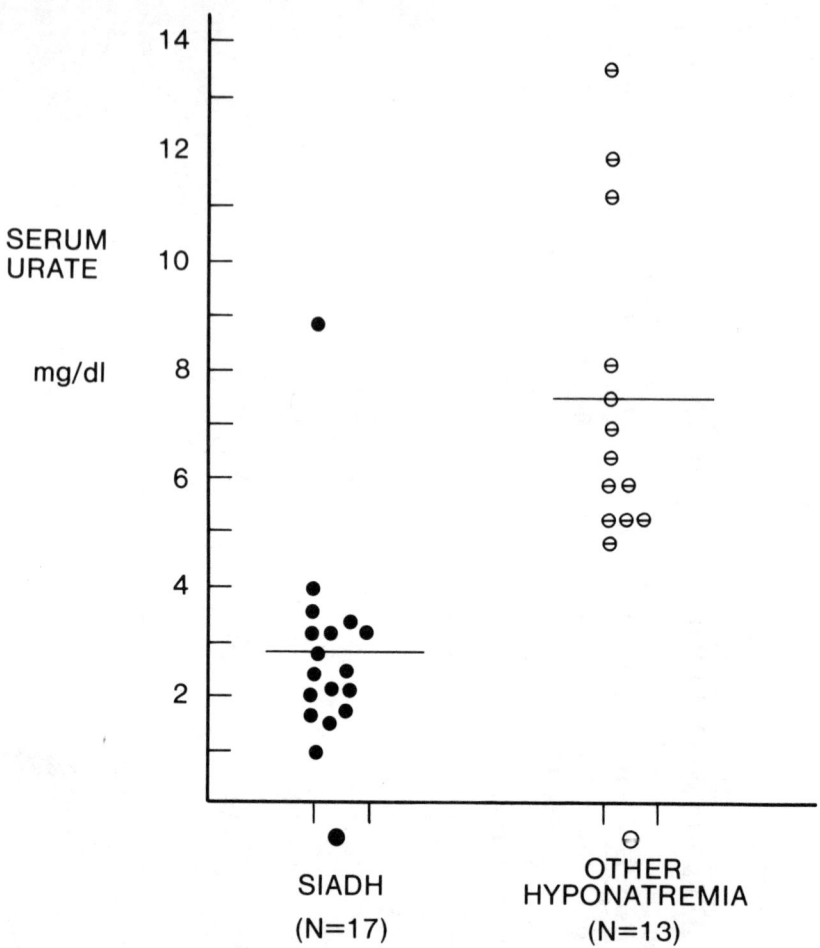

Serum concentrations of urate in each patient during hyponatremia.

L. Rhabdomyolysis Presenting as a Metabolic Derangement

A 24 year-old white female is brought to the Emanuel Hospital Emergency Department after three days of vomiting, diarrhea, and flu-like symptoms, including myalgia and malaise. She has a cardiac arrest (asystole) in the ambulance on the way to the ER and is promptly resuscitated with epinephrine 1:1000 .5 cc in 10 cc NS IV and 1 amp $CaCl_2$. The ERB-18 reveals an increased anion gap and Ca = 6.2 mg/100 ml, PO_4 = 11.4, and Mg = 2.8. The constellation of hyperphosphatemia and hypocalcemia (without renal failure) suggested the presence of rhabdomyolysis. CPK measured 224,000 units. Patient was given mannitol diuresis but expired the next day after several bouts of EM dissociation secondary to hypocalcemia.

COMMENT: Elevated PO_4 and low Ca can be caused by acute rhabdomyolysis or renal failure.

M. Ethylene Glycol Ingestion

A 22 year-old white female is brought to the St. Vincent's Hospital ER in a delirious state. The patient was accompanied by her brother who stated she had been drinking beer in the back seat of a car but had accidentally opened a can of break fluid and ingested an unknown amount. On physical exam the patient had irregular respirations (rate = 12), HR = 120, T = 37.2, BP = 95/60. The patient was intubated and an ETOH drip (½ mg/kg) was started. The ERB revealed: Na = 139, Cl = 98, HCO_3 = 20, K = 4.6, BUN = 12, Cr = .9. An ETOH level (prior to the drip) = 120 mg percent. Measured serum osmolality = 332; calculated serum osmolality $(2 \times Na + BUN/3 + Glu/20)$ = 286. Urinalysis was WNL, without calcium oxalate crystaluria.

COMMENT: The differential between measured and calculated serum osmolality = 46 mosm. An ETOH level of 120 mg percent will account for only about (120/4.5) 26 osm, suggesting the presence of a substance with osmotic properties (i.e., polyethylene glycols) that will also account for an anion gap of 21.

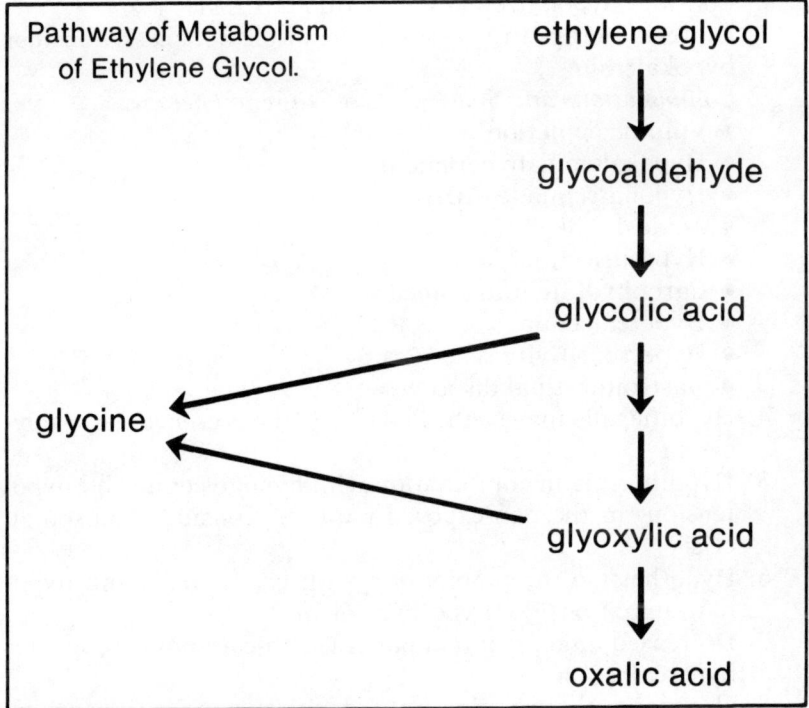

Pathway of metabolism of ethylene glycol.

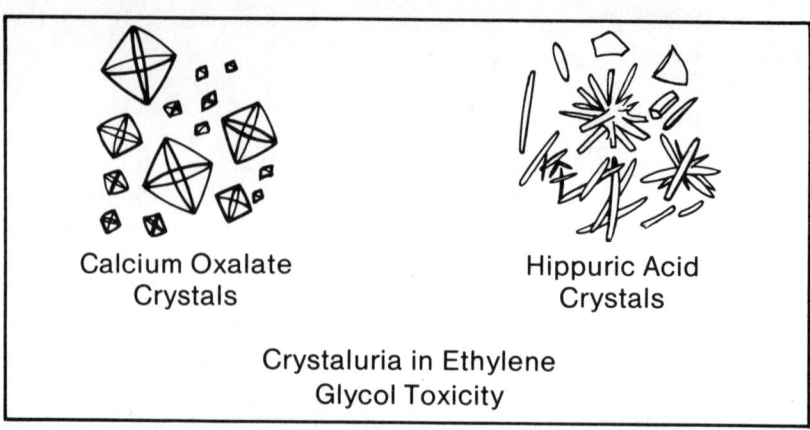

Calcium Oxalate
Crystals

Hippuric Acid
Crystals

Crystaluria in Ethylene
Glycol Toxicity

Crystaluria in ethylene glycol toxicity.

VII. SOME "CLINICAL PEARLS" FOR METABOLIC EMERGENCIES

1. Refractory ventricular fibrillation: Consider hypokalemia
2. Diuretic therapy in a patient with altered mental status: Consider hyponatremia with/without SIADH
3. Diuretic therapy in a patient with muscle weakness: Consider hypokalemia

   Complications and Side Effects of Diuretic Therapy
   - Volume depletion
   - Hypokalemia, hyperkalemia
   - Hyponatremia (SIADH)
   - Acidosis, alkalosis
   - Hyperuricemia
   - Carbohydrate intolerance
   - Hypercalcemia
   - Hypersensitivity reactions
   - Gastrointestinal disorders
4. Hypothermia may be the first clue to the presence of hypoglycemia
5. Hypothermia in combination with hypoglycemia and hypotension (in the non-exposed patient): Consider Addisonian crisis
6. Hypothermia in combination with bradycardia and hyponatremia: Consider hypothyroidism
7. Decreased anion gap in a patient with carcinoma: Consider hypercalcemia
8. Hyperphosphatemia in a patient with shock: Consider superimposed lactic acidosis

9. Hypocalcemia, hyperphosphatemia, and hyperuricemia in a patient with crush injury, muscle aches, or after strenuous exercise: Consider rhabdomyolysis
10. Increased anion gap in a patient with elevated serum osmolality: Consider ETOH ketoacidosis, ethylene glycol, methanol, or paraldehyde ingestion
11. Focal neurological lesions in the diabetic: Consider both nonketotic hyperosmolar states and hypoglycemia
12. Acidosis and hypercapnia in patients with COPD: Remember the acidosis may represent an underlying and potentially correctable *metabolic acidosis*—you have to look for it!
13. Unexplained symptom complex consisting of neurological, hematological (thrombocytopenia, decreased O_2 delivery by RBCs, etc.), cardiac (cardiomyopathy), and/or respiratory (failure) disturbances in ETOH abusers, diabetics, and starved individuals: Consider hypophosphatemia

REFERENCES

HYPEROSMOLAR HYPERGLYCENIC NONKETOTIC COMA

Arieff AI, Carroll HJ: Cerebral edema and depression of sensorium in non-ketotic hyperosmolar coma. Diabetes, Vol 23, p 525, 1974

ALCOHOLIC KETOACIDOSIS

Hamburger S, Rush D: Alcoholic ketoacidosis—A review of 30 cases. Jour Amer Med Womens Assoc, Vol 37, p 106, 1982

Fulop M, Hoberman HD: Alcoholic ketosis. Diabetes, Vol 24, p 785, 1975

Berl T, Anderson RJ, McDonald KM, Schrier RW: Clinical disorders of water metabolism. Kid. Int., Vol 10, pp 117–132, 1976

Harrington JT, Cohen JJ: Clinical disorders of urine concentration and dilution. Arch. Int. Med. Vol 131, pp 810–825, 1973

Ross EJ, Christie SBM: Hypernatremia. Medicine. Vol 48, No 6, pp 441–473, 1969

DIABETIC KETOACIDOSIS

Kreisberg RA: Diabetic ketoacidosis: New concepts and trends in pathogenesis and treatment. Ann Intern Med, Vol 88, p 681, 1978

INDEX